Genetics, The Fetus and Our Future

Carmel Bagness
MA (Medical Ethics)
RGN, RM, ADM, PGCEA

Published by Hochland and Hochland Ltd, 174a Ashley Road, Hale, Cheshire, WA15 9SF, England.

© 1998, Carmel Bagness

First edition

ISBN 1-898507-65-1

British Library Cataloguing in Publication Data
A catalogue record for this book is available from the British Library

Printed in Great Britain by Cromwell Press Ltd.

Contents

Acknowledgements

I would like to take this opportunity to express my deepest gratitude to my husband, Mike, for his understanding and encouragement during the composition of this piece of work.

These thanks are additionally extended to family and colleagues.

Table of Cases

Acts of Parliament

CHAPTER ONE

Genetic Engineering and Our Future

Introduction

In recent decades the embryo and fetus have come under considerable scrutiny from a variety of sources. Knowledge and understanding of physical development has led to a greater appreciation of environmental, social and genetic effects on the developing fetus (the term fetus is used to include embryo, unless embryo is mentioned specifically). This greater awareness has created controversy, especially in relation to the moral and legal status of the fetus, where discussion is concerned with potential or real rights and responsibilities towards this developing human being. Historically the moral status appears to vary with the demands of a particular society and, generally speaking, the moral position has had some effect on any legal standing the fetus may appear to have had, although it has also been influenced by other factors.

The most recent, and possibly most controversial evolution of knowledge is with regard to the human genome (i.e. the total number of genes in the human cell). At present the identity and purpose of individual genes is not fully understood, and it is believed that there are between 50,000–200,000 genes in the human genome (Weatherall, 1991). Molecular biologists across the globe are working on projects attempting to identify and map the entire genome (Kevles and Hood, 1993). Such knowledge may provide the answers to a greater understanding of the capacities and limitations of human beings. This may be achieved by finding potential solutions to inherited diseases and some claim that it may also offer the opportunity to alter potential traits in others (Kevles and Hood, 1993).

The whole concept of genome mapping and the subsequent use of the knowledge is vast and will potentially affect all aspects of human living. It involves various disciplines including molecular science, genetics, all areas of health care, sociology, educational programmes, ethical and legal matters. The particular interest herein lies in the analysis of the ethical and legal effects of such knowledge on the embryo and fetus. This is in part due to the recent legislation regulating embryo research (Human Fertilization and Embryology Act (HF&E), 1990) and the variety of media coverage – both factual and sensationalist – surrounding genome information and genetic

1

engineering. Current text does not allow the opportunity to consider in depth the developments in molecular biology which are creating these new and exciting possibilities, therefore the main focus of attention will be on the moral and legal issues relating to the fetus. This chapter will provide an introduction to the progress of the Human Genome Project and an outline of the concept of genetic engineering. This exploration will also include discussion about genetic disease and genetic manipulation, as this would appear to be the main focus of attention for the embryo and fetus in the future.

The remaining chapters will focus on discussion and analysis of the moral and legal status of the fetus. Ethical issues appear to be related to the concept of personhood, and when, or if, the fetus becomes a person. This, in turn, leads to a variety of moral issues involving what could or should be done to a fetus who is incapable of consenting to any procedures or therapies imposed on him.[1] It will also involve consideration of recent developments in embryo experimentation and how gametes (the collective term used for the ovum and sperm) have been treated in law. It would appear that moral views tend to inform any legislation that may be seen to regulate and 'protect' the fetus, and though they may be closely linked, they do not always appear to be compatible.

The moral and legal status of the fetus is changeable and can vary within societies, therefore discussion will include an historical perspective as well as focusing on current practice, with some analysis of future possibilities. The practical application of genome information in the form of genetic engineering is an exciting subject, as are the ethical and legal questions invited from such a potential breakthrough in the greater understanding of who we are and how we really function (Dixon, 1993). This will also involve some discussion about the issues surrounding infertility treatments, as they will probably form part of the process to be developed. One such question (or series of questions) lies in the future ethical and legal status of the fetus. If scientists are able to produce a fetus according to parental or societal specification, will the fetus and embryo have any moral status, or will they simply be seen as a series of cells undeserving of any 'human' rights or other forms of protection? Or will he be viewed as a *better* human being than his ancestors?

---

1. The author acknowledges that fetus and embryo may be male or female but for the purposes of convenient reading they will be referred to in masculine terms within the text.

The human genome discoveries

The nucleus is the largest structure within the human cell, is responsible for the control of cellular activity, and contains the genetic information. The genes are molecules, which are packaged into 23 pairs of chromosomes, and are made up of Deoxyribonucleic Acid (DNA), whose specific structure allows both copying and division of the genes (Tortora and Grabowski, 1993). The main function of genes is in determining the structure of peptide chains, which are strings of amino acids that form the building blocks of enzymes and other proteins (Weatherall, 1991).

Human cells produce a variety of proteins:

a) structural proteins which help form plasma membrane and other parts of the cell;
b) functional proteins which can serve such diverse functions as hormones, antibodies and contractile elements in muscle tissue (Van De Graaff and Fox, 1989).

The instructions for making these proteins are found in the DNA, and the cells produce them by transcription and translation of the genetic information encoded in the DNA (Tortora and Grabowski, 1993). Genes are a vital component in sustaining life, but their specific functions have not yet unfolded. Some 4,500 genes have been identified to date (Rennie, 1994). However a daunting task lies ahead for those who choose to identify the remainder, some 50,000–200,000 (Weatherall, 1991), with this estimate varying according to different sources, Judson (1993) suggesting a figure of 50,000.

Many authors (including Kevles and Hood, 1993; Weatherall, 1991; Emery and Mueller, 1992) place the beginning of the process with the re-discovery of Mendel's Law of Inheritance in the 1900s, which was followed throughout the first half of this century with various scientists improving on his theories and ideas. The next landmark was in 1953 when Crick and Watson described their double helix model for the structure of DNA (cited in Kevles and Hood, 1993). This discovery appears to be the cornerstone of the current surge of interest in the genome, although the idea of mapping it did not take root until 1984. Those brave or curious enough to try are now working on various Human Genome Projects throughout the world, involving scientists from the USA, Japan, Britain, Italy, France, Russia and many other interested countries – an international alliance to develop knowledge. The co-ordinating body for these projects is known as HUGO – Human Genome Organization (Hawkes, 1994). In 1990 James Watson (cited in Caskey, 1993) wrote that the genome project will have a description of the human genetic map within 15 to 20 years!

The driving force behind the projects are:

1.   the search for knowledge of what each gene is responsible for,
2.   how genes functions,
3.   how each gene may be affected by other genes (Blackburn and Loper, 1992).

The primary purpose of HUGO is to develop an accurate and complete map (including sequencing, the process of determining the order of an individual's nucleotides on a fragment of chromosome) of all, or most, of the human genes. It is not concerned with finding solutions for defective genes – genetics (Fig. 1.1) and genetic engineering will hopefully fulfil this role.

The study of genetics is concerned with two issues:

a) how traits of anatomy, physiology and behaviour are inherited;
b) how each individual expresses those traits in their development, both in utero and throughout life (Judson, 1993, p. 37).

Fig. 1.1

Identifying each gene will not complete the exercise – it is estimated that only three per cent of all diseases are carried by single gene defects (Rennie, 1994). The more complex conditions (e.g. heart disease and cancers) involve a host of genes which can affect a person's predisposition to develop an illness. It is also important to acknowledge that genes are not totally responsible for the development of these illnesses, as environment, upbringing and a host of other circumstances also contribute to susceptibility to genetic diseases. Rennie (1994) also remarks that it is estimated that everyone carries at least five to ten genes that could make them ill under the wrong circumstances or could adversely affect their children. A solemn reminder is included, 'we are all mutants… everyone is genetically defective' (Rennie, 1994, p. 69).

Gene mapping determines the relative positions of genes on the chromosomes, and the distance or proximity of two or more genes. According to Judson (1993) the belief is that the closer together genes are, the less chance there is of them being separated during meiosis and hence the greater the probability that they will be inherited together.

HUGO's ultimate goal is to know how genes contribute to the vast array of human characteristics and the role they play (or do not play) in disease, development and behaviour. This knowledge will undoubtedly revolutionize current thinking on human development of normal characteristics, such as organ function, and abnormal ones, such as disease states. It may ultimately enable us to enhance or prevent our physical and behavioural genetic fates (Kevles and Hood, 1993).

The main focus for medicine would appear to be increasing the knowledge base about the aetiology of disease by identifying those genes responsible for inherited disorders such as Cystic Fibrosis, Huntington's Chorea or Alzheimer's Disease. It is also becoming clear that many diseases, previously considered not to be genetically linked (like heart disease and some forms of cancer), may have a genetic link. Once the sequence has been identified, the focus of attention can turn to possible treatment or prevention. Health promotion may take on a whole new meaning in the light of these discoveries, in particular pre conception care.

The ethical concerns raised by knowing adult or child genetic profiles are vast and as such will only be mentioned here, as current discussion is concerned with the fetus and embryo.

For the adult, the potential of knowing such information may work towards them enjoying life and taking appropriate measures to ensure comfort and a reasonable standard of living. This may be true if they know they are at risk of developing a debilitating disease, but Greely (1993) warns that there are potential discriminatory issues which need to be addressed. Concern is raised with regard to issues of employer's rights to know an employee's genetic profile, which could affect job prospects, education, insurance cover and a variety of health and safety issues. It also calls in to question the whole issue of access to profiles, for example should future partners have access, or insurance companies etc?

Knowledge of child profiles may well influence the relationship with the parents and other family members. This may be positive or negative and may not just be in terms of psychological interactions. It could include life choices being made for them in relation to education, health and life style.

Rennie (1994) also brings up the issue of defining abnormality, suggesting that in a health conscious, aesthetically dominated society, traits such as baldness and obesity may be 'abnormal' or 'undesirable'. This may have major significance when (if) it becomes possible to choose desirable or acceptable traits. The term eugenics appears frequently when reading about developments in the Human Genome Project, which prompts concerns about attempting to produce a perfect race. The word *eugenics* (from the Greek root *'good in birth'* or *'noble in heredity'*) was first used by Francis Galton (cited in Kevles and Hood, 1993) in the late 1880s, when he proposed that the human race might be improved (as with plants and animals) by selective breeding to produce only the best. It would appear that his ideas became popular, especially among 'white, middle and upper-class professionals' (Kevles and Hood, 1993, p. 5) until the 1930s when the term was also associated with Hitler's notion of how to create this perfect race.

However, the idea of perfection is tantalizing to many, the idea of perfect people who only enjoy the best of life seems particularly appealing. It is fair to say that many believe in modified versions of this concept – those concerned with the elimination of disease and relieving pain and suffering. The outcome may be to enable more people to be capable of fulfilling a 'useful' life within a successful society – whatever that may be defined as! If this is voiced as a possible future, what of the fate of the embryo? Will parents go to any lengths to *attempt* to have perfect babies?

Once the human genome has been mapped and sequenced, the focus of attention will then turn to appropriate use of the information. The legal and ethical issues raised will create controversy about access to information, confidentiality, consent to treatment, experimentation and research, ownership of information and the morality of a society who may have within its grasp the unprecedented ability to change the course of human development, for better or worse.

Genetic engineering – the answer to our dreams!

In 1973 scientists developed techniques whereby they could alter the instructions provided by the genes in bacteria. They discovered that by adding genes from another organism to bacteria, it caused the bacteria to produce proteins that they would not normally synthesize – this DNA which comes from a variety of sources is called Recombinant DNA and the new technology was referred to as genetic engineering (Tortora and Grabowski, 1993). *Genetic engineering* is a blanket term covering technologies such as gene therapy, gene manipulation, modification, cloning, recombinant DNA technologies and 'the new genetics'. This new technique opened up developments in plants and animals beyond the dreams of science prior to this discovery, but it is not without controversy, especially in relation to its potential use on human beings. Nicholl (1994) suggests that there are three main areas where such technology is valuable:

- basic research on gene structure and function;
- production of useful proteins by novel methods;
- generation of transgenic plants and animals.

Genetic engineering has been used with relative success in plants and animals for some time now. Dixon (1993) suggests that there were over 62,000 animals with new genetic codes born in British laboratories alone in 1991. These advances have encouraged scientists to further the technology to include human subjects, hence the search for the human genome information. Current text does not allow elaboration on the issues concerning plants and animals, however a brief explanation of how the technology works may provide an understanding of what could be achieved when the secrets of genes are unlocked.

Emery and Mueller (1992) provide an overview of the steps in the technology (also see Nicholl's book (1994) for further details):

1. **Restriction Enzyme Cutting which generates DNA fragments in such a way that a particular gene or segment will be included**
    In order to add to or alter genes, techniques had to be devised whereby specific genes or segments of DNA could be removed. In 1970 Smith (cited in Emery and Mueller, 1992) discovered that certain enzymes of bacteria had the ability to cut DNA. Each one is designated according to the organism from which it was derived and the type of fragment that a particular enzyme produces will depend on the recognition of the gene sequence and on the location of the cutting site within that particular sequence (Nicholl, 1994).

2. **Incorporating the DNA fragments into a suitable carrier**
    Once the gene/s or DNA segments have been removed they are incorporated or cloned into a suitable carrier. DNA ligase (a cellular enzyme) is used to join the Recombinant DNA molecules. The ability to cut and join DNA molecules provides the opportunity to create recombinant DNA within a test tube.

3. **Transformation of the host organism**
    After the foreign DNA has been incorporated into the vector, it is introduced into the host by transformation, which is the method of making the plasma membrane of the cell permeable to the vector. There are a variety of methods used, such as exposing the bacteria to calcium salts, which create sufficient permeability to allow entry to the cell (Emery and Mueller, 1992).

4. **Cloning**
    Cloning is the process whereby large quantities of a particular DNA sequence are produced (Nicholl, 1994). This is achieved by growing the host vector in a bacterium to produce multiple identical copies of the individual recombinant DNA molecules that have been generated.

5. **Selection of clones containing the relevant DNA fragments**
    Finally the appropriate clones must be selected. Once a particular DNA fragment has been cloned, it is then possible to determine the order of an individual's nucleotides on that fragment. This is known as sequencing.

Once genes have been isolated and the appropriate clones selected, it then becomes possible to contemplate gene manipulation, in vivo (within the body) as well as in vitro (in a test tube or similar external mediums). In the future, genetic engineering techniques may make it possible to clone the zygote, whereby the 'original' fertilized ovum and sperm would be implanted, while the clones could be frozen as 'spare part' embryos for the future should the original individual develop organ failure or another disease necessitating 'replacement parts' (this point will be elaborated on in Chapter 4). Work with fetal tissue transplants suggest that it may be possible to use one of the cloned embryo's to graft to the original. Ferguson (1990) explains that research on fetal tissue transplantation to adults suggests that the fetal tissue will lose some of their histo-compatibility transplantation antigen, which significantly decreases the risk of rejection.

However he goes on to explain that the maximum number of clones possible from a single embryo would be about four (because of the nature of cell division in the early embryo), making such projects both non economically viable and impractical. The alternative would be to develop a 'communal bank of transplantation antigen free cells for use by everyone' (Ferguson, 1990, p. 18). The cells would be derived from IVF procedures and would be available to the population as a whole rather than just those who had a cloned embryo in storage. However such procedures are futuristic and as such will not, at present, impinge on any realistically orientated discussion about the effects of genetic engineering on the moral and legal status of the embryo.

Currently, genetic engineering techniques involve embryo experimentation and if developed further will involve considerable risk to the human embryo, which may also involve tissue transplantation.

Embryo research and tissue transplantation

In the late 1970s the fertilization of the human egg in vitro made it technically possible to observe and actively research the early developing embryo. Research has since advanced in two different directions, and it is necessary to explain the distinction between the two, because of the outcomes for the embryo.

The first is *life enhancing research*, which is carried out in the hope of improving the life of a particular fetus or embryo, and can be conducted anytime during pregnancy with the mother's permission. They include fetal surgery and medicine which is still in a somewhat experimental phase, but appears to be having phenomenal success. This includes advances being made in intra uterine blood transfusions, surgical repair of obstructive opathies, repair of diaphragmatic hernia, intra-uterine bone marrow transplants and conversion of fetal arrhythmia's (Schenker, 1992).

The second type, *life threatening research*, is the one concerned with in this discussion and can only be conducted up to 14 days gestation, is regulated by the HF&E Act (1990) and will (at present) lead directly or indirectly to the death of the fetus and embryo.

Allowing such research would appear to disregard any special status these human entities have either for their potential to become moral thinking beings or simply because of their humanness.

At present embryos for research come from two sources:

1. *Spare embryos* are so called because they are left over from IVF treatments. The argument justifying their use is that provided the mother's permission has been sought (and there appears to be some dispute about this point), then some scientists believe that it is better to put them to use rather that simply discard them, which is what would happen anyway (Glover et al., 1989).

2. *Research embryos* which are created from donated sperm and ova and fertilized specifically for research. There appears to be more controversy over the idea of creating embryos just for research purposes, as it disregards any serious notion of human 'rights' or special status by creating a human being just to experiment on and destroy before he has the opportunity to fulfil his potential.

In conducting such research, scientists appear to be disregarding any moral status for these embryos. However, can the potential advantages to be achieved from such research significantly outweigh the loss of some embryo?

This research has led to developments in:

a) Contraceptive facilities, which is seen by many as a vital role in population control and safer motherhood, for those who can choose (e.g. an attempt is underway to develop an anti-sperm antibody vaccine for use as a contraceptive).
b) Understanding, diagnosis and treatment of infertility (by providing information of the mechanisms involved in the hope of improving existing procedures and introducing new ones for the treatment of infertility that is at present untreatable).
c) Advances in the treatment of miscarriage and ectopic pregnancies. It is now believed that a large percentage of miscarriages are due to implantation defects or embryonic abnormalities, therefore studying the development of the embryo may lead to methods of treatment for women who suffer recurrent miscarriage; it may also help in understanding why ectopic pregnancies occur.

d) Detection and understanding of genetic and congenital abnormalities (embryo biopsy, Dawson, 1993).

e) Fetal Tissue Transplantation (Ferguson, 1990). If this innovation continues to maintain its current apparent success, it may lead to treatments for Parkinson's Disease, diabetes and other abnormalities.

With regard to detecting abnormalities, a procedure known as embryo biopsy has been conducted on primates and mouse pre embryo. It involves removing one or two cells from the four or eight cell pre embryo and growing them in a culture for examination and possible manipulation (Dawson, 1993), while the remaining cells are frozen until the results are known. This then provides an option of which embryo to implant in the uterus. However, the success rates for Gamete Intra Fallopian Tube transfer (GIFT) remain low in humans so this only remains a possibility for the future. Dawson (1993) stresses that further research is needed, especially into embryo freezing and detection of abnormal genes, before such treatments could be used clinically.

The other area of advance in relation to embryo research is that of the use of fetal tissue for transplantation. Ferguson (1990) reports on the current developments in the use of embryo and fetal tissue and cell transplants, where experiments on animals and humans have shown some success. The cells/tissue are currently taken from embryo and fetus who have been spontaneously or therapeutically aborted and does not involve in vitro techniques. However it would be theoretically possible to derive embryos from in vitro fertilization and allow them to develop until they are required for transplantation. The main reasons for continuing to develop these processes appear to be:

1. Fetal cells and tissue possess an unprecedented capacity for colonizing, invading and differentiating in adult organs. It seems possible that by grafting fetal tissue to existing adult organs (rather than replacing them) they are capable of taking over the functioning of the defective organ.

    As there is a major shortage of suitable donor organs, this could lead to a significant decrease in suffering and death for many (Ferguson, 1990).

2. Research has also demonstrated that early embryos grown in vitro appear to lose some of their histo-compatibility transplantation antigens, which decreases the likelihood of being rejected by the recipient (Ferguson, 1990).

Having established the value of transplantation research, there are two options as to how they could be used:

a) embryo/fetus to adult
b) embryo/fetus to embryo/fetus.

EMBRYO/FETUS TO ADULT
With regard to adults, there are two methods which have been used with some success in trials.

i)   Introduction of hormone secreting cells to colonize a particular gland where the existing cells were either malfunctioning or have been destroyed. The diseases most likely for such therapy include diabetes and thyroid dysfunction (Ferguson, 1990). In 1993, Begley et al. reported that in 1987 a team of immunologists, in the USA, transplanted fetal pancreatic tissue into 16 people who suffered with Juvenile Onset Diabetes. In all cases the tissue '...insinuated itself into the patients tissue, differentiated into the islet cells that churn out insulin and survived' (Begley et al., 1993, p. 50).

ii)   The second possibility involves grafting tissue to existing organs to restore some function, for example, using embryonic nervous tissue to restore neuro transmitter function in particular areas of the adult brain (Ferguson, 1990). In 1992, Fletcher reported on current research using such methods to relieve the symptoms of Parkinson's Disease, suggesting that although they are still researching the techniques, the outcomes appear favourable.

EMBRYO/FETUS TO EMBRYO/FETUS
Ferguson (1990) reports that animal studies have shown positive results of transplants between donor and recipient fetus, suggesting that donor tissue should be added to enhance functioning of a defective organ rather than replacing it. The advantage of fetal transplantation over adult is that the fetus can grow to accommodate the extra tissue easier than an adult could. Again the donated tissue could be derived from aborted fetus or in vitro prepared embryo, which returns the discussion to whether such therapies/ research should be allowed.

The arguments against embryo research rest largely on the moral status of the embryo and fetus. Does society have the right to use these embryos simply as a means to an end? Glover et al. (1989) suggests that some scientists believe that if they are spare (left over from IVF treatments), then it is justifiable to use them rather than just destroy them unused, but should they be created in the first place, and what of embryos deliberately created for research? Conservative thinkers would probably object to either, as there can be no justification in creating or using human embryos and then destroying them for the benefit of others. Such a policy gives little value to their potential to become moral persons or their human uniqueness.

Higginson (1987) argued the case against research on the basis of natural justice, that it is intrinsically wrong to treat embryos simply as a means to an end. His argument, that if society exercises logic, coolly and compassionately, then there is a duty to offer the same protection to embryo's as adults:

> 'Many substantial benefits might occur from performing lethal experiments on you and me, but our precious dignity as human beings would have been terminally violated in the process. We are fortunate enough to be able to seek shelter under the Helsinki Declaration, and in particular the provision that the interests of science and society should never take precedence over considerations relating to the well-being of the human subject.' (Higginson, 1987, p. 40)

As embryo research is ongoing it appears that the benefits have outweighed the concerns about the embryo and future therapies may be seen in a similar light.

Genetic disease and genetic manipulation in human beings

Today, medicine is continually attempting to improve the health and well-being of society. This is achieved, partly, by a greater understanding of disease states and partly by using the ever more efficient technology to produce treatments or plan health promotion programmes.

Genetic disease is responsible for significant mortality and morbidity worldwide. According to Braude (1992), there are over 4,000 diseases caused by a single defect and many more thousands are inherited on a multifactorial basis.

The human genome project hopes to access these links, but before moving on to future possibilities, it is necessary to consider that which is currently available to those affected. There are no known treatments for many genetic disorders, however for some there are options available (Braude, 1992):

- Metabolic manipulation: Some genetic diseases are caused by a failure to function, or lack of, a specific enzyme activity, therefore dietary restriction may be all that is needed to control the negative aspects of the disease. For example, phenyketonuria can be successfully controlled following diagnosis, by a reduction in the intake of phenylalanine.
- Replacement of a gene product: Some disorders are caused by the lack of a product of a gene and this can be administered to the person to overcome the deficiency. For example, insulin in diabetes or clotting factor in haemophilia.
- Tissue transplantation: In some disorders it may be possible/necessary to replace organs which are not functioning normally.

For example, some success has been reported with cystic fibrosis sufferers where heart-lung transplants has helped overcome the deteriorating lung function.

Knowing the cause of an illness and the pattern of its inheritance goes some way towards finding treatments or preventable measures. However the gap between cause and treatment is vast and medicine will have to attempt to keep up with the human genome project to avoid a disappointed society, who may know why they are ill but can do little about it.

Genetic modification

For some diseases, *gene therapy* is a potential answer. This would involve the insertion of genetic material directly into cells (to alter, delete or repair genes), which would positively affect the functioning of the cell and hopefully correct the genetic defect. The procedure is outlined in Figure 1.2.

The sequence of events necessary for gene therapy are:

1. The gene responsible for the defect must be isolated and cloned (this is already underway with HUGO);
2. An appropriate carrier cell for the gene must be selected and the required gene has to be inserted into this carrier (Microbiologists are currently working on techniques for the insertion of genes (Nicholl, DST 1994);
3. Once the gene has been inserted, the cell must continue to reproduce and function normally, including the new gene producing the required product (Braude, 1992).

Fig. 1.2

Caskey (1993) suggests that the most promising agent for this procedure could be the retrovirus. Once a retrovirus infects a host cell, it makes a DNA copy of its RNA (genetic material of retroviruses is RNA not DNA), and this DNA is integrated into the chromosomal DNA of the cell during the normal life cycle of the virus.

Braude (1992) explains that the virus is modified:

1. to contain the defective or deficient protein; and
2. so that it is unable to replicate itself after entering the host.

Once inserted (usually via micro injection into the nucleus of the cell), the cell produces messenger RNA from the new sequence, which will then code for the defective or deficient protein. This sounds simple enough, however it is not without side effects. There is always the danger that the virus may undergo spontaneous mutation and begin to replicate itself, creating a new disease state within the individual, or it might transform the cell into a carcinogenous state (Braude, 1992).

Somatic or germ line cell gene therapy

Such therapy would have differing results whether one uses *somatic cells* (cells of the body), or *germ line cells* (reproductive cells). If *somatic cells* are used the individual is the only one affected. For the adult, somatic cell gene therapy holds similar ethical questions as for someone undergoing major surgery, for example informed consent, autonomy, and confidentiality, as well as issues of risk:benefit ratio. The argument being that any advantage or disadvantage sustained will be limited to that person and is unlikely to affect any offspring or future generations (Watt, 1993). This is assumed but factually it is an unknown entity at this present time.

The other issue in relation to somatic cell line therapy is that of enhancement and eugenic genetics, which is considered to cause greater ethical concern. French Anderson (1990) defines these two concepts separately, whereas many authors appear to use the terms interchangeably. The distinction made is thus:

> *Enhancement Genetic Engineering*: '...involves the insertion of a gene to try to "enhance" a known characteristic; for example, the placing of an additional growth hormone into a normal child.'

> *Eugenic Genetic Engineering*: '...an attempt to alter or improve complex human traits each of which is coded by a large number of genes; for example, personality, intelligence, character, formation of body organs.' (French Anderson, 1990, p. 147)

He states that such eugenic therapy is purely theoretical and is, from a practical viewpoint, impossible for the foreseeable future. However the story is quite different with enhancement therapy, although the practical issues are formidable. The idea, to date, with gene therapy has been that of replacing defective genes, 'Fix the broken part and the human machine should operate correctly again' (French Anderson, 1990, p. 159). However there is a significant danger that if one inserts a gene in the hope of improving or selectively altering a known characteristic, it could potentially alter the metabolic balance of the entire body, therefore a great deal more research is needed before enhancement therapy becomes available.

With regard to the fetus and embryo, such therapy could be conducted with the fully informed consent of the mother *and* provided it is to prevent a major defect or debilitating disease developing, it can hold few ethical concerns. The issue is somewhat different when the techniques become possible for other traits and characteristics, such as hair/eye colour, stature or some complex characteristics, such as behaviour and intelligence. Where can the line be drawn? If a woman wants to alter the genetic makeup of her future child with safe technology, that could make him taller or thinner than would be expected, should she be 'allowed' to do so? What counselling etc. will be available to guide her autonomous decision? The issue of her autonomous decision is an entire ethical debate of its own, as consideration has to be given to the whole issue of who will be 'allowed' to make decisions and choices – parents, clinicians or someone else?

The issue of *germ line cell therapy* is much more contentious, as the intention would be to alter genes in such a way that any modifications would be passed from one generation to another. This therapy involves the insertion of the replacement gene into the reproductive cells of an individual, which means that the alterations (desired and undesired) would be created in subsequent generations. This would involve not only inserting the gene into the right cell, but also ensuring that it would be transmitted safely to the next generation. However, if successful, it could be an efficient way of removing genetic diseases from society. Notwithstanding that, Watt (1993) reports that animal studies on germ line therapy have demonstrated a worrying increase in abnormalities and death in the subjects being studied, without even contemplating the possible problems in future generations. Again this is futuristic therapy but deserves discussion from an ethical standpoint because it may become technically possible. Annas and Elias (1993) also suggest that it should not be totally dismissed because it may prove to be the only way to effectively treat some diseases.

There are two potential processes for achieving germ line therapy, both considered by most authors to be futuristic at present (French Anderson, 1990; Braude, 1992):

1. **Genetic modification of early stage embryos**
   Using this technique, early developing embryos are fertilized in vitro, genetically altered (by inserting genes, repairing defective genes or deleting genes) and then implanted into the uterus.

   This is considered to be the more viable of the two options even though it involves in vitro fertilization (IVF) and considerable risk to the embryo.

2. **Genetic modification of the parental germ cells**
   This process involves altering the genome of the parents germ cells (involving therapy on the unfertilized ovum or sperm). Thereafter the altered germ cells should produce genetically altered gametes.

There is of course no guarantee that other genes may not become defective during gametogenesis and fertilization, which makes this the less realistic option, apart from the practical issues of accessing the sperm and ovum.

However, if the procedure is possible with somatic cells and the technology available, will such techniques be prevented by society? Would society demand access to such possibilities, looking only at the short term issues and not taking on board possible long term consequences? What of the fate of the human cells/young embryo that such therapies may be carried out on?

Society is going to have to decide whether germ line gene therapies (which has been described by Nicholl (1993) as akin to changing the gene pool) can safely and effectively produce the desired effects without side effects in successive generations. 'Testing' such therapies on human beings could take many generations to determine all the possible effects and the use of animal studies (even if permissible) may not produce accurate results.

Braude (1992) also has reservations about the practicalities of modifying germ line cells themselves but he does concede that current technology is improving daily, so the future may make these visions possible.

Will genetic manipulation alter personal identity?

Another area of concern is that of identity. If genes contain the total inheritance package of an individual, and gene therapy alters some of those genes, does that person still exist? Elliott (1993) and Persson (1995) both discuss the issue of causing a new individual to exist and an 'old' one to cease to exist. Elliott (1993) argues that because the amount of genetic material being changed is so small, it would not cause disruption to individual identity. Persson (1995) progresses the argument to state that even if genetic therapy did affect identity, there could be 'person regarding reasons' for conducting it, for existence can be better than non existence for the individual.

Another issue that is of concern is whether people with Recombinant DNA (i.e. DNA from a variety of sources) could be viewed as less than human. However the aforementioned arguments can be used to refute such a notion, on the basis that the minute amount used could be compared to the use of implants today (e.g. hip replacement), and these people are still regarded as 'whole' human beings.

The alternative to germ line or embryo therapy would be an attempt to eliminate potential genetic disease carriers or affected individuals by gamete or embryo selection. This could be achieved either by only selecting 'fit' embryos for implantation, or by post implantation selection through prenatal diagnosis and subsequent termination of the pregnancy, or selective feticide in cases of more than one live embryo. Again who is to decide what a fit embryo is, and there are no guarantees that further abnormalities will not develop after implantation or later in pregnancy. This alternative will create issues related to the abortion debate and right to life, as well as issues of maternal rights and autonomy.

Conclusion

The Human Genome Project is a reality, gene mapping and sequencing is under way and time *appears* to be the only barrier to obtaining genetic profiles, in the same way as it is now feasible to obtain blood profiles. The potential effects of knowing one's capacities and limitations will span all aspects of human life from conception (or before) to adulthood. Those involved are excited by these developments. However having information is one issue, but its utility is quite a different matter and it raises many concerns for society as a whole.

Anyone who has contact with people who suffer from disabilities caused by inherited disorders will appreciate the need for the advances made to enable better treatment and/or prevention. However, as with many advances there is the 'slippery slope' concern of how far one will go to relieving or eliminating a disability. Antenatal screening for fetal abnormality is currently being carried out to access the chromosome map of a fetus and the future holds more sophisticated methods of predicting health and lifestyle through genetic profiling. The more that is known about genes, the more predictions can be made.

The question is how far will it go? The possibility of fetal genetic profiling is becoming more real, which creates the concern that it may leave parents with the option to terminate a pregnancy where the fetus is affected by, or predisposed to, an inherited disease because there is no treatment available. Or will they have the option of deciding to have the genes altered or replaced using genetic engineering? If this becomes possible, and all indications are that it will, how many genes will it be possible to replace? Through engineering it may become possible to replace more than one defective gene, how will parents decide which ones to alter if their fetus is shown to be predisposed to several 'undesirable' abnormalities? This may also depend on how abnormality will be defined! Will it include obesity, which can be fatal, or baldness, which can cause severe depression in some? One has to then consider the eugenics option – could this be used to produce the 'perfect baby' – a tall blue-eyed, male, Caucasian, vegetarian, intellectual or whatever the desired 'perfect person' will be at that time? Or will parents settle for children who will be *lucky* enough not to develop debilitating diseases?

Even if such genetic therapy will not be available for many years it may not be acceptable to many, who would for a variety of reasons (as with abortion) reject the idea of manipulating their fetus. On the other hand, there is a danger of increasing the number of pregnancy terminations following knowledge of genetic profiling. If the profile does not match parental expectations, or shows an increased risk (under certain circumstances) of a potential adult disease developing, will that fetus be at risk of being terminated? Whatever the future, careful counselling and advice will need to be available for parents who may choose to go down that particular road.

There are also issues of 'who will be in control of these potential parenting issues, will it be parents, obstetricians or scientists?'. Authors such as Stanworth (1987) are already concerned about the mechanization of motherhood, where the real decisions about parenting no longer lie with parents but are held by the technology used. Women may have demanded access to safer techniques to control fertility and their birth experiences, as well as the outcomes of their pregnancies. However Stanworth (1987) suggests that women's demands only play a small part in the agenda driving the technological developments,

> 'For obstetricians and gynaecologists, specific types of reproductive technologies may carry advantages quite separate from their impact on mothers and infants. Reproductive technologies often enhance the status of medical professionals and increase the funds they can command, by underpinning claims of specialised knowledge and by providing the basis for an extension of service.' (Stanworth, 1987, p. 13)

This leads on to another issue, that of cost, which will not be considered here in detail but will need to be on future agendas. Suffice to say that consideration will have to be made whether these therapies will remain in the private sector, or whether demand will force them into the public health care arena, possibly putting further strains on current limited resources.

The aim of this particular exploration is to analyse the potential effects of the human genome knowledge and the effects of genetic engineering on the fetus. The term 'eugenics' appears regularly and causes concern, not least because of the chequered history that the word evokes. The notion that genetic engineering may have the capacity to produce perfect babies has already been muted to society via the media, using headlines such as:

> 'We now have the means to select the baby of our choice' (Pilkington, *The Guardian*, 1st January 1994)

'How to tell Frankenstein the yuk stops here' (Oddie, *The Times*, 9th January 1994).

The interesting point in all this is that no one appears to have described 'the perfect baby' – there are so many variables for perfection – race, intelligence, height, weight, to mention but a few. Who could set the criteria for perfection or normality? Or will we become more tolerant of differences when we truly know ourselves and our genes! In relation to the embryo and fetus, one has to raise concerns about their role in the developments in genetic engineering. As already explained gene therapy is not without risks, is it morally and legally acceptable to experiment on human embryos, knowing the potential risks? Or do the potential advantages significantly outweigh the disadvantages? Many of the possible answers involve our current thinking on the moral and legal status of the fetus, and it is from this perspective that the author intends to begin.

Chapter 2 will focus on the moral status of the fetus, in an attempt to come to some consensus on the validity of differing claims over when the fetus becomes a person and should, as such, be treated with a respect equal to that status. This discussion will also contemplate the theory of potential personhood, which adds another dimension to this rather complex issue.

Currently, legislation allows experimentation on the embryo up to 14 days. However one of the main concerns with HUGO developments is whether it will change the legal standing of the embryo in relation to experimentation and treatment. Even if the 14 day limit is retained, that may already allow alterations to the genetic makeup of the embryo, so consideration may have to be given to possible changes in legislation. Chapter 3 hopes to explore and analyse the past and present legal status of the embryo and fetus, in an attempt to understand how legislation focuses, or not, on fetal rights.

Chapter 4 will provide some analysis of current ethical issues, and legal problems which may manifest themselves in the future with genetic engineering techniques. Will the aim be towards the elimination of debilitating diseases or will it be the dawn of a new era of eugenics? As these treatments will almost certainly involve some of the infertility treatments currently in use, Chapter 5 will focus on some of the issues surrounding these therapies, with particular reference to the status of the embryo. Chapter 6 will focus on the future of the embryo and fetus and, due to the unprecedented nature of the knowledge being developed, this will involve some speculation during which it is hoped to evoke some discussion and possibly an answer to the question as to whether the Human Genome Knowledge Explosion will affect the moral and legal status of the embryo and fetus in the future?

CHAPTER TWO

The Moral Status of the Embryo And Fetus

Introduction

The central issue behind questions relating to what 'ought' or 'ought not' be done to the embryo and fetus lies in their claim to a moral status, that is having some moral significance comparable with children or even adults. Many of the debates about 'right to life', 'quality and/or sanctity of life' rely heavily on one's belief about when life begins to matter morally, and why human life is considered so valuable.

It is largely agreed that human beings have a moral awareness, which is one possible criteria for when one becomes a person. The development of moral awareness in an individual will, to some extent, depend on the circumstances of their life and the environment they live in, although some (Fulford et al., 1994) argue that it may be an innate part of development. Urmson (1994) looks in depth at how we actually arrive at our moral code, considering whether it is something that we have discovered over the centuries (that some forms of behaviour are favoured over others) or that it is some form of pure thought discovery, like seeing the necessity of mathematical truths. He also suggests that it may be simply something that we have invented, for whatever reason, because we find it desirable to do so. The question of the moral status of the fetus appears to be less concerned with moral awareness and has more to do with when society believes a life holds moral significance. This leads one to consider why life is seen as valuable.

What attributes do humans have that make them significantly different to fish, animals or trees? When considering the value of life, most authors make the distinction between life and personhood. Life, being the physical existence of a 'being', recognizable as a member of the species Homo Sapiens, whereas personhood is the personal identity, which has moral significance – the 'human' part. White (1994, p. 337) suggests that personhood involves mental processes, and it is intrinsically linked to our understanding of physical developments in the embryo and fetus, '...the greater the gestational age of the fetus, the more developed are the characteristics of personhood, or perhaps our own ability to recognize them'. Gillon (1991) states that a minimal condition for this personhood is a capacity for consciousness or sentience; whilst for others it is necessary to be self conscious and self aware (Tooley, 1972).

The main intention here is to explore the various opinions on the moral status of the embryo and fetus. This involves identifying the concept of moral significance and focusing on just when that status is meaningful enough to allow for consideration of interests and rights. This is particularly important today with the advances being made with Human Genome Organization (HUGO). Diversity exists as to when life and personhood begin, and many have endeavoured to draw lines at different stages of development in attempts to determine when life begins to matter morally.

These 'line drawers' appear to fall into three broad categories:

- **the extreme conservative** – who believes that life begins at conception;
- **the moderate view** – who believe that life/personhood begins during the intrauterine period. This view is often associated with the time when the fetus has potential viability; viability being a state when the fetus can survive outside the uterus, i.e. without physiological support from the mother (J.T Noonan, 1991);
- **the extreme liberal** – who believes that personhood begins at or after birth.

The extreme conservative view is usually categorical, as will be demonstrated. The latter two groups provide a variety of views and for this reason they will be discussed together, as they both argue that life and personhood begin at different stages of development.

This chapter will focus on the different theories used to defend or defeat the aforementioned categories. It begins by looking at two concepts of the human being – biological and moral. This will be followed by a brief (as it largely appears to be accepted) discussion on the issue of the existence of moral significance. The inclusion of such an overview was felt necessary as any claim to moral significance by the fetus and embryo derives from a prior claim that human beings have moral significance.

The main discussion concentrates on the issues of life and personhood, focusing on the theories used to decide just when, or if, the embryo and fetus develop personhood status. This will also include consideration of the theory of potential personhood, and an examination of the moral status of genes, as they are the building blocks of human life, when confined to their gametes.

The human being

When considering the human being and 'its' significance within the universe, there are three concepts to contemplate:

- the biological being;
- the legal status (which will be covered in Chapter 3);
- the moral significance.

Biologically, it can be argued that life potentially begins with oogenesis and spermatogenesis, continuing with fertilization, zygote development, implantation and fetal development. Life can be traced further through childhood, adolescence, adulthood, old age and on to death. This continuum can be traced using technology, and as such it is possible to demonstrate the existence of life at the earliest stages of development. There are some who argue that life begins with Gametogenesis (the synthesis and production of the ovum and spermatozoon) (see White, 1994) but the majority appear to accept that it begins at fertilization. However, the current discussion is not so much concerned with when human life actually begins to exist but with when it holds moral significance, and this appears to occur at or sometime after fertilization.

At this point it is necessary to elaborate on the boundary dividing the embryo from the fetus. *Fetus* is the term used to describe the developing human being from six weeks gestation to the time of birth. The definition of the *embryo* is a little more complex. Until fairly recently, the embryo would have been defined as the developing human being from conception to six weeks gestation. However, Moore (1983) states that the embryo commences some eight days after fertilization, which is when the blastocyst (the early developing fertilized ovum) defines its cells into an inner cell mass and the embryonic disc appears. In 1989 McLaran (cited in Jones and Telfer, 1995) suggested the use of the term *pre embryo* to describe the 'entire products of the fertilized egg up to the end of the implantation stage' (McLaran cited in Jones and Telfer, 1995, p. 32), which is usually completed by the end of the second week of gestation, with the appearance of the primitive streak at about 15 days.

The primitive streak, which appears as a series of cells at one end of the embryonic disc, is *considered to be* the first recognizable feature of an embryo (Warnock, 1985). However it should be noted that many other experts in the field do not use this term and refer to the term embryo. The legal justification for use of the term pre embryo appears to be ethical in origin, referring again to the personhood arguments. The controversy appears to be less about whether the pre embryo is a human being and more to do with the notion that it has not yet become an *individual* human being.

Many texts continue to use the term embryo for development from fertilization to six weeks, although it should be noted that this distinction does have some significance in personhood arguments. The controversy arises with the knowledge that until the primitive streak appears, twins or higher multiples of embryo may develop any time up to this point, therefore these cells do not constitute an individual human being. It can be argued that using such a term denies the existence of the potential human being from conception and may provide a plausible excuse for allowing research on this entity (Holland, 1990) because it could not be legally protected (Morgan and Lee, 1991).

The early developing cells also divide to produce the embryo and the placenta, so the argument goes, if one is to treat the pre embryo with personhood status should one treat the placenta with similar significance? As the placenta does not carry any of the components alluded to for personal identity it is unlikely to attain any personhood status, and consequently it seems easy to dismiss such an argument. However that still leaves the status of the so called pre embryo.

The human being and moral significance

There appears to be an assumption that because we value human life it does have moral significance. It also seems reasonable to argue that our existence demonstrates some value, as issues of killing and injuring others are largely prohibited, except in times of war, where moral issues of survival appear to overtake those of killing and injuring.

There are a variety of moral positions to support the claim to moral significance, and Gillon (1991, p. 42) suggests four principles which confer moral obligation between human beings, and are particularly relevant to medical ethics:

1. **All sentient beings are morally equivalent**
    i.e. beings that can experience pleasure and pain.
    Bentham (cited in Gillon, 1991) argues that suffering is more important than reasoning in terms of moral significance but his claims include animals as well as humans, because of their ability to feel pain and experience pleasure.

2. **Membership of the species Homo Sapiens** confers the moral importance that all living and innocent human beings have a right to life.

3. **All viable human beings have this right to life**, however as will be demonstrated later, viability appears to be a movable event.

23

4. **Being sentient also means possessing special attributes grounding the unique moral importance due to people, including their right to life.**

However, there are reasonable arguments to counter all of these claims, for example, being a member of the species Homo Sapiens may simply be explained as speciesism (Gillon, 1985). Speciesism is a term used by Singer (Gillon, 1985) which suggests that moral status in human beings is simply related to our needs (moral or otherwise) to positively discriminate towards our own species – Homo Sapiens. There are those who argue that we should not be species specific, and that some animals may acquire similar status, depending on our definition of personhood. Singer (cited in Gillon, 1985) claims that human beings tend to have many interests that most animals do not and cannot have, for example, an ability to be self aware and plan for the future, as well as attributes such as the capacity for abstract thought and complex communication. However, as Gillon (1985) points out, some animals may have those attributes. Warnock (cited in Gillon, 1985) does not have a problem – she appears to accept that we have every right to be species specific by the very nature of our humanness.

Finnis (1973) and J.T. Noonan (1991) both proposed that because the products of a human conception are the result of human parents with moral values, this gives the embryo moral significance, but those who believe that life and personhood begin at different stages may not agree with this perspective.

Life and personhood

The key issue appears to be that of making a distinction between human life and personhood. Through modern technology it is now possible to demonstrate how life begins at conception and progresses through a developmental continuum which will, if successful, eventually lead to an adult life.

It must be acknowledged that this process is fraught with problems and it is only if the formation is successful, that the zygote will become an adult. Assessing and determining the point at which this being becomes an individual with a personal identity of 'its' own is more complicated. However before discussing the various personhood theories, it is necessary to consider the concept itself.

What is personhood?

Personhood is an important concept, especially in relation to the embryo and fetus, because its existence will acknowledge acceptable or non acceptable practices in terms of treatment, research and a right to life. It has been defined simply as the right to be accepted as a member of the species Homo Sapiens, but involving more than just physical resemblance and genetic similarity, as suggested by Gillon (1991).

Warren (1991) refers to this concept as moral humanity, as opposed to genetic humanity, that is being a 'fully fledged member of the moral community'. In her argument against the 'right' of the fetus to be a person, she discusses five principles necessary for personhood, although she does concede that an entity does not need to possess them all to be considered a 'proper' person. It is in this concession that perhaps her argument is counter productive. Her principles are:

1. **Consciousness**
    of objects and events external and/or internal to the being, and in particular the capacity to feel pain;

2. **Reasoning**
    the developed capacity to solve new and relatively complex problems;

3. **Self-motivated activity**
    activity which is relatively independent of either genetic or direct external control;

4. **Capacity to communicate**
    by whatever means possible;

5. **Presence of self concepts and self awareness**
    either individual or racial, or both (Warren, 1991. p. 440).

It is possible to counter her argument in favour of the fetus. For example, in relation to consciousness, the fetus can respond to touch, noise and other external and internal stimulus (J.T. Noonan, 1991). Other philosophers have put forward variations on these principles, however they all appear to include the above as significant elements in relation to defining a personhood status. The focus usually returns to notions of consciousness, reasoning and self awareness. However, the interest here is more on when personhood does develop, which appears to be just as complex as that of determining what the concept means.

When does personhood develop?

Rumbold (1993) suggests that all those who remonstrate about when personhood begins fall into two categories:

a)   those who believe that life and personhood begin at conception;
b)   those who believe that life and personhood develop separately and at differing times.

LIFE AND PERSONHOOD BEGIN AT CONCEPTION

The first group, usually religious believers but not exclusively so, have faith in a form of divine power and accept that a human being has three facets: body, mind and soul/spirit. Even this point is disputed in that Christians and Jews believe that only people have souls, whereas Hindus and Jains believe all animals also have souls (Pojman, 1992).

This standpoint, religious or not, is categorical, insisting that the most important essential of these is the soul/spirit. It is considered to be infinite and exists from the beginning of life (Rumbold, 1993). Even if the body is deformed or the mind unbalanced, the soul/spirit lives on even past death of the body, and so it is inviolable. The belief is that the soul is our true self, that which gives us worth and it becomes disassociated from the body at death and continues to exist. Pojman (1992) reminds us that many questions remain as to the existence of the soul, however for those who do believe in this concept, the answer to when life becomes morally significant would seem fairly straightforward.

Life and personhood are part of the same continuum, so the embryo and fetus should be treated with equal respect and rights because of the existence of the soul/spirit. Having this viewpoint would mean that experimentation on embryos, some infertility treatments, and some forms of contraception would not be morally acceptable. It would also prohibit any intentional injury or death. This suggests that it may even reject gene therapy completely.

This standpoint is also taken by those who believe that life is important from conception because of the potential of the embryo to become an adult, which will be discussed later.

LIFE AND PERSONHOOD DEVELOP SEPARATELY

The second group (the moderate and extreme liberal view) believe that life and personhood develop separately and that the human being is made up of body and mind. Both groups define their particular boundaries differently:

Viability as a boundary

Moderate thinkers usually focus on the time of viability as being the beginning of personhood. This argument often involves the notion that dependence on another human being forms a basis for denying any personhood status. Using viability as a time when the fetus can become independent of the mother has its own problems, because this independence is purely physiological, and newborn human babies remain dependent on others for successful growth and development for some time after birth.

The other issue with using viability as a boundary is that it is also a 'movable feast'. At present a fetus is considered viable from 24 weeks gestation following the HF&E Act (Morgan and Lee, 1991). However the potential for developing technology to bridge the gap between in vitro embryo and incubated babies cannot be dismissed as fiction. J.T. Noonan (1991) suggests that such technology is only a matter of time and so independent viability cannot be considered an absolute time for development of personhood.

Focusing on the other end of the life continuum, Glover (1990, p. 124) also reminds us that if we use 'potential physical independence as a necessary condition' for personhood we may create further dilemmas, where perhaps a time may come when dependence (temporarily) on another human beings organ may cause a redefinition of viability. J.T Noonan (1991, p. 435) reports that different racial groups have different viability limits, in particular, '... Negro fetuses mature more quickly that white fetuses. If viability is the norm, the standard would vary with race and many individual circumstances' such as weight and height!

The sharpness of boundaries is arbitrary. Viability was considered to be 28 weeks up until the HF&E Act 1990 (Morgan and Lee, 1991), and in time the current 24 week limit may recede to 22, 20, 18 weeks or below. Historically, other boundaries have been used, such as quickening (a term used to describe the first fetal movements as felt by the mother, usually around 14–16 weeks gestation) as it was traditionally regarded as the first signs of a live fetus, and definite confirmation of the pregnancy.

Birth and beyond as a boundary

The other boundary currently aspired to is the birth of the baby. This is an apparently sharp boundary, when the fetus becomes a baby and is accepted as having a personality of his own. However, one has to wonder whether this is used out of sentiment of recognizing a vulnerable 'miniature person' rather than any identifiable principles involving onset of personhood. Recent research on parents' perception of their pregnancy, when viewed on ultrasound, suggest that this could change if the fetus were visible to all '... a majority of women interviewed... valued ultrasonography in early pregnancy because it confirmed the reality of the baby for them' (Neilson and Grant, 1991, p. 432).

Birth as a boundary may be a convenient line to draw because of the attractions of the baby existing. However there is little to suggest that the adaptation from fetus to newborn baby bestows any special moral significance that can be argued objectively.

There are also those who argue that personhood does not develop until sometime after birth. Tooley (1972) contends that one '... possesses a serious right to life only if [one] possesses the concept of self as a continuing subject of experiences and other mental states, and believes that [one] is [one]self such a continuing entity'. He goes on to suggest that this state does not develop until sometime after birth but appears somewhat reluctant to suggest that a week after birth is a useful boundary. However he is leaving the details to psychologists to establish just when a newborn baby comes to believe that he is a continuing subject of experiences and other mental states.

Whichever boundary is used, both moderate and extreme liberals believe that personhood and life begin separately and their arguments are based on the belief that the human person is made up of a body and a mind. Discussion has already established that the human body can be verified from conception. However with regard to the mind, this second group usually argue that if the mind has not begun to function or no longer has the capacity for rational thought then 'it' is no longer a person (Rumbold, 1993). The argument then lies with defining when the mind begins to function and stops functioning. One major concern with this idea is that if one loses one's ability for rational thought (perhaps temporarily – under anaesthetic or in a comatose state) then one is no longer a person or deserving of any special rights that personhood bestows! The extension of this principle is when death occurs. Death used to be measured on a biological level – with cessation of vital organ function, whereas now the focus is more on brain death. Pojman (1993) discusses the brain orientated concept of death, suggesting that the absence of brain function equates with the '... absence of the possibility of personal life... the person is dead' (Pojman, 1993, p. 114). So when does the brain begin to function?

The beginning and development of the mind, contained within the brain, appears to be rather elusive to define. The physical development of the nervous system, of which the brain is a part, is a continuous process. It is believed to commence with the appearance of the primitive streak, around the second week of gestation (Moore, 1983). By day 17 the neural groove appears, followed by neural folds, which fuse and form a recognizable antecedent of the spinal cord (Warnock, 1985). However this does not allow us to understand when consciousness begins, which is considered to be the foundation of other necessary attributes such as reasoning and rational thought (Jones, 1989) and one of the hallmarks of personhood. Jones goes on to suggest that consciousness begins when differential brain activity occurs, which is said to be about 40 days after fertilization. However, he states that brain activity, demonstrated using an electroencephalogram, may be as late as 24–28 weeks gestation (Jones, 1989). He also concludes with scepticism about the usefulness of such information in relation to determining personhood. Therefore one has to consider other mental processes which may be significant in determining when personhood commences, if not at conception.

Tooley (1972) argues that self awareness is a necessary feature of being a person (in the morally important sense of having a right to life), and he goes on to state that in order to have rights, one must have an ability to recognize what a right is. As the fetus is not self aware, he can have no right to life. Tooley extends this argument to include infants and attempts to justify infanticide as being morally permissible. He defends this position on the basis that people prefer to have and raise 'normal' rather than 'handicapped' children, and '... if it could be shown that there is no moral objection to infanticide, the happiness of society could be significantly and justifiably increased'. His argument is further developed by suggesting that infanticide is a taboo subject rather than one with rational moral prohibitions.

Notwithstanding this utilitarian view, the fact remains that there are deeply felt intuitions about infants having a moral status that bestows on them a right to life. There is also some concern here of sitting on 'the slippery slope' – that once some individuals (possibly children with severe learning disabilities, who cannot recognize what it is to have a right) are deprived of their right to life, other infants and/or adults may be at risk, if they are no longer seen as 'useful, whole persons' – however that may be defined.

Another point that is relevant here is the issue of sanctity of life versus quality of life. 'The Sanctity of Life Principle' argues that all human beings have a right to life and killing or deliberately injuring is wrong, whereas the 'Quality of Life Principle' concerns itself with the person doing more that mere living.

Pojman (1992) states that the two are opposed on the basis that life should be about reflection and moral deliberation to be a life worth living. From this, it may be surmised that the arguments about development of personhood includes those of quality of life, or do they? The conservative viewpoint would appear to suggest that all life is sacred and therefore deserving of rights and privileges, partly because of its potential to become a self aware, rational being. The extreme liberal viewpoint may argue for a certain quality for life, before admitting some human beings to 'personhood status'. However, finding some common criteria for this 'quality' issue may prove too elusive, as individual perception of 'quality' varies enormously.

When is a person a person?

Glover (1989) states that being a person may not have sharp boundaries. Just as there is no single moment when one enters middle age, there is no definite line drawn at when one develops the distinctive characteristics of personhood. It would appear that attempts by philosophers to determine the characteristics of a person prove too diverse for consensus. Some, as we have seen, identify with the presence of life, while others (Gillon, 1985; Warren, 1991) suggest that it involves an ability to reason, to self determinate and be self aware. Dennett (cited in Glover et al., 1989) proposes that it involves a sense of justice and Tooley (1972) suggested that personhood begins when one can recognize what it is to have a right, although they did not have to be able to communicate that understanding.

Harris (1992:18) states that '... a person will be any being capable of valuing its own existence'. He explains that the value of life is not necessarily quantifiable because people are so diverse: that what one may value as important may be different to what another may believe. He suggests that it is not the particular reasons for valuing life that are important, but the simpler fact that if a person values their life then it should be seen as valuable. It can be reasoned from this that it is wrong to kill a person because in so doing, one would deprive that individual of something they value – their life.

If one attempts to 'test' the aforementioned characteristics in relation to the fetus, difficulties arise in assessing ability to reason or to be autonomous. The fetus does not have the ability to value his life, therefore he is not in a position to be morally offended if injured or if that life is taken. The extreme liberal view could include infants and children as well as those who suffer with severe learning disabilities – who may never develop an ability for rational thought or self awareness.

This position may also include those at the other end of the life spectrum, who have lost their ability to reason through illness or accident – would they be persons? According to some of the principles used, probably not, yet we do value this life at present. However one has to consider that the arguments being used in favour of euthanasia may well change this position of value in the future.

In reality, at present we do treat these groups with respect and they are afforded 'rights' and because we do, it is then possible to swing the arguments towards the fetus, on the grounds that the embryo and fetus are potential persons and should be treated with respect; because they may become autonomous beings.

The potential person

The main defence for arguing that a fetus is a person lies in the fact that embryonic, fetal and infant development is a biological continuum and to draw a line at a specific time in that process is arbitrary. It is also noteworthy that all the genetic material for personhood exists from conception. Therefore does having the potential for personhood equate with having the rights of personhood?

Thompson (1971) argued that it does not follow that because one has the potential for something, that it should have automatic right to the privileges of that status. She uses an analogy of an acorn – being an acorn does not equate with being an oak tree. Another comparison could be that of having the potential to be an Olympic Gold Medal winner. Having the potential would not give that individual the right to the privileges that go with such an accolade before winning. However, one is not concerned with oak trees or accolades here but with something much more valuable – human life.

It is relevant here to focus on the notion of value, in terms of human life, as Harris writes (1992, p. 9) '... when we ask what makes human life valuable, we are trying to identify those features, whatever they are, which both incline us, and entitle us, to value ourselves and one another, and which licence our belief that we are more valuable (and not just to ourselves) than animals, fish or plants'. The value of personhood appears relative to those deciding when identity begins to develop. H. Noonan (1991) provides extensive discussion on theories relating to personal identity, suggesting that it is closely linked with our responsibility for past actions – our experiences and responses are the things that keep us motivated and emotional about life and living. He proposes that our pasts and futures are the primary focus of many of our central emotions and attributes. He would appear to be suggesting that in order to have a personal identity, one needs a past, with experiences to focus on. As the fetus has no known past, it would be difficult to argue that he has a personal identity. However, J.T. Noonan (1991) argues that even the embryo at eight weeks gestation is responsive to touch, and so at that early stage is at least experiencing, whilst the zygote is certainly alive and responding to its environment.

Poplawski and Gillett (1991) reason for the consideration of a relative sanctity for all human life, that even if a person does not have an intrinsic right to life, the fact remains that the life form exists from conception and few people would prefer if they had never existed. Becoming a person is a progressive evolution of stages linked by development. Their argument is that each stage is an essential component of the whole, it is not feasible to draw a line at any one stage: 'At one stage of this whole, the individual becomes a rational social being and an inherent moral value is realized. We then take this moral value, inherent to human beings, as rational social beings (persons) and attach it to the form as a whole' (Poplawski and Gillett, 1991, p. 62)

The moral status of genes and gametes

Genes are the building blocks of human beings, and therefore discussion about the moral status of the embryo and fetus, raises questions about the moral status of genes and subsequently gametes.

If the embryo/fetus is a potential person and as such should be treated with a respect due to all persons, is it not unreasonable to suggest that gametes are potential persons? The sperm and ova carry the genetic material necessary for human beings to survive and become persons, so should they not be treated in a similar way? Steinbock (1992) suggests that if this were the case then contraceptive practices would be viewed as wrong, 'In using a spermicide, one commits mass murder!' (Steinbock, 1992, p. 63).

However, those who might agree with the concept of potentiality appear to disagree with such notions on the basis that there is an enormous difference in probabilities when it comes to whether one sperm or one ovum will result in an adult (one in two hundred million for the sperm and somewhat less for the ovum), compared with an 80 per cent chance of zygotes succeeding beyond birth (Noonan, cited in Steinbock, 1992). (Current research on miscarriage suggests that this percentage may be more like 50 per cent (Oakley et al., 1990) or less. Murphy (1992) suggests that as many as 1:5 pregnancies may end in miscarriage.) Either way the odds for survival are dramatically increased once sperm and ovum survive together.

Steinbock (1992) further demonstrates this point by referring to Warner, who argues that, 'All things being equal, the zygote will grow into a person. On the other hand the ovum or sperm itself is neither growing nor developing no matter in what sort of environment one should find it or put it into. A gamete will not, by itself, grow into anything other than what it already is' (Warner cited in Steinbock 1992, p. 64). If one accepts this apparently widely held view (Warnock, 1987) then it can also be deduced that gametes, while separate, are not potential persons and as such research, experimentation and therapy does not cause moral dilemmas – provided they remain unfertilized.

Parthenogenesis is a naturally occuring phenomenon, whereby the ovum can be stimulated to grow without fertilization and produce female embryo. It is also now possible to induce parthenogenic growth in vitro.

Harris (1993) argues that it is possible that the human egg is an individual member of the human species as it contains all that is necessary for continuous growth to maturity under the right conditions. However Johnson (cited in Harris, 1993) states that these female embryo do not survive once the heart beat becomes apparent. He believes that this is related to the absence of '... the required activity in the placenta of the paternally imprinted chromosomes from the father'.

However, Harris (1992) speculated that if this technicality could be overcome, then it may be possible to produce an all female race, with no help from the male population! He discusses this subject at length, and concludes that it is unlikely to be technically possible, and '... the chances of all women uniting on any issue, let alone... on an issue of an all female world, may be remote' (Harris, 1992, p.173). It is also reasonable to argue that such a choice would be undesirable for a variety of reasons, which will not be explored here.

Warnock (1987) also discussed the relevance of human cells having rights and argued that the issue of the embryo having rights can be divorced from the question of personhood, and concluded that the nature of the humanness of the human embryo gives it a special status and as such it should be treated differently.

Conclusion

The moral status of the fetus varies, as with all moral issues, a perplexity of views exist. Once one accepts that human life has moral significance, the next issue is to determine when the embryo and fetus deserve some moral recognition and as such 'personhood rights'.

It would appear to depend on how people see their own moral status. Some see it as instruction from God, while others see it as some set of rules debated upon and laid down by society, and often constructed to reduce conflict (e.g. killing, stealing, causing harm to people is morally wrong). The whole issue of acquisition of moral significance appears to be parallel with, but not reducible to, the answer to 'when does "one" become a person?'

If one believes in divine power, life and personhood begin at conception, and the embryo and fetus who survive beyond that should be treated with respect, and his position as a potential person gives him a right to life and some personhood status.

At the other end of the debate, there are those who believe that life is merely a set of cells functioning biologically, and their significance is only in their ability to contain a person, at some time. The extreme liberal believes that this person develops at or after birth, and is deemed a person when they possess a concept of self as a continuing entity.

In the middle of the debate one finds a significant body of thinkers who believe that personhood begins when the fetus becomes viable. Viability appears to be a movable concept. Steinbock (1992) suggests that the development of an artificial placenta would also rule out this notion of viability being important for personhood status and some authors suggest that the pre implanted (extra uterine) embryo is viable because it can survive outside the woman's body – time and technology being the only barriers to extra-uterine incubation for the whole gestation. Currently, viability is put at 24 weeks gestation, but this is not a fixed concept with the advances made in neonatal medicine and technology.

This discussion focuses on the views held by society in relation to the issue of just what, *if any*, moral significance we should bestow on the embryo and fetus. What must be remembered is that living in a pluralist society demonstrates divergent and consequently conflicting moral principles, hence the debate here and elsewhere.

Glover (1990) proposes that moral principles are 'tested' by our acceptable or non acceptable responses to their consequences. Society is currently having to respond to issues involving harvesting ovum from aborted fetuses and post menopausal pregnancy due to the advances in science. In the near future, issues of genetic manipulation and other techniques will be items for debate. This will again highlight the disagreements about moral status and what can or should be allowed to happen to another human – whether he is acknowledged as a person or not. Recent media reports, on the advances in genetic engineering in plants and animals, have a high profile (Kohn, 1994; Hawkes, 1994), and appear to create prolific discussion about the acceptability and usefulness of such techniques. It will be interesting to 'watch this space' when the reports and discussions focus on 'human subjects/genes'.

From the previous text, it has been demonstrated that there are opposing views as to when the embryo and fetus become a person. Both Pro life and Pro choice lobbies are vocal and increasing in number and strength, which suggests that society as a whole has not yet decided on this complicated issue. It is questionable as to whether one answer is possible within such a pluralist society. This may mean that such decisions can only be resolved through legislation, which should reflect a balanced and supportive view of all members of the society. This point may be debatable if based on the outcome of the Abortion Act in 1967, as since then a significant section of society continue to fight for their rights and the 'rights of the unborn'. However legislation does have a significant part to play in what may or may not happen to embryos and fetus, both today and in the future. The subsequent chapter will focus on this legal status, taking a historical and present day perspective, with a view to an analysis of the possibilities for the future.

CHAPTER THREE

Legal Issues: The Status Of The Embryo And Fetus Past And Present

Introduction

Ethical values and legal issues can be seen as quite separate and distinctly independent of one another even though they are both concerned with concepts such as rights, responsibilities and justice. A law is legally binding whereas a moral code may create an opportunity to critique that law. It should be noted, at this point, that the author acknowledges that the law is different in various countries across the globe and that it is morally underpinned in some more than others. Historically, moral concerns have been reflected in legislation e.g. murder is a crime, and legal frameworks have often led to more tolerant views of moral behaviour (as a result of the Wolfenden Report, 1957, society may have become more tolerant of homosexuals (Downie and Calman, 1994).

The intention of this chapter is to explore the historical and current day perspectives of the legal status of the fetus in both common and statute law, with a view to contemplating the possibilities for the future of the human genome. It appears that in the past the focus on legislation has been in relation to property rights (inheritance and ownership) and to the right to life (abortion law). Curiously, the fetus has been treated quite differently when dealing with these issues. More recently, reproductive technology has added a new dimension to the way society and legal institutions view the fetus, in particular in relation to the embryo. For example, the developments in genetic engineering have created new, possibly unprecedented questions relating to ownership of gametes and the obligations, or not, that society may have towards their protection.

In order to consider this legal status the interaction between legal and moral rights will be explored, as archival evidence suggests that they are linked. It also demonstrates that the legal status appears to have created an equal measure of controversy. The fetus cannot presently exist successfully outside of the mother before 24 weeks gestation (except in vitro, following extra uterine fertilization, but this is presently limited to 10–14 days gestation). Therefore any legal status it may or may not have has to be balanced with the rights of the mother, and this may inevitably create conflict for some women: In common law the fetus has no legal personality, with any rights only maturing after birth, although historically and currently, the fetus is afforded some protection, if only indirectly in relation to the mother.

It becomes apparent that different areas of the law come to quite diverse conclusions about any legal status the fetus may have. Gentles (1990), referring to the 'grotesque contradictions' of a legal system, states that:

> '... the unborn child enjoys the right to inherit property; she can sue for injuries inflicted while in the womb; and she has the right to be protected from abuse or neglect by the mother. On the other hand, she no longer enjoys... the right not to be killed.' (p. 147)

The following explores this apparent contradiction, while discussing the 'rights' 'enjoyed' by the fetus, who, by the nature of his existence within the mother (or a test-tube) is not capable of having interests of his own until after birth – by which time the damage may be done.

The quotation by Gentles (1990) prompts for a definition of right, and just what is meant by having rights? It is acknowledged that English law is not determined in terms of rights as such and any reference to rights is a focus on moral rights, such as the right to life. Glover (1990) defines moral rights as being 'absolutes; they may not be infringed, however great the advantages of doing so'. Notwithstanding his argument about these rights being absolute, the whole issue of ethical debate concerns itself with deciding what is or is not a right and so even that (the right to life) is not absolute, as will be demonstrated.

It should be noted at this point that the law is usually involved when problems arise and as such deals with a minority of cases, the exception to this being the law pertaining to abortion, which deals with a significant number of 'cases'. The majority of children may not need to invoke or enforce rights, based on the assumption that their parents will protect them and care for them from conception to a time when they can look after themselves.

The fetus, property laws and the law of tort
The fetus and property law
Historically, the fetus seems to have 'enjoyed' various levels of legal status and this appears to have been strongest in relation to property laws. Grisez (1970) provides a comprehensive summary of how the fetus has been compared to the child in legal cases involving inheritance of property. In fact, in the Earl of Bedford's case (1586 4 Coke 7f7 [1586] – cited in Grisez,

1970) the fetus is referred to as a child. In this, and several documented cases, provision for the heir's children included those which were *'pars viscerum matris* – part of the mother's insides'* (Grisez, 1970, p. 362). She goes on to argue that the real purpose of such laws was less to do with the rights of the fetus and more to do with the provision of continuity of ownership of property and titles.

The fetus and the law of tort

This notion is further explored in Tort Law (torts being civil wrongs, done by one person to another), where any legal status appears to have been ignored. In order to bring an action the wrong doer and the wronged party must be in existence, which reverts to the issue of personhood and the existence or not of the fetus as a person. A precedent was established in 1883 (in the USA) in the Dietrich *v.* Northampton case ([1884] 138 Mass. 14 (USA) cited in Grisez, 1970) that an unborn child was not a person. The case involved a claim for prenatal injuries by a woman who had suffered a fall and miscarried. The child lived for 10–15 minutes after birth, but Justice O.W. Holmes ruled that the non-viable unborn child was not a person (Yates and Yates, 1992).

A further case in Ireland in 1891, Walker *v.* Railway Co. (28 L R Ir. 69 [1891]) added to this non person idea when Justice Johnson asserted that: '... when the act of negligence occurred the plaintiff was not esse – was not a person, or a passenger, or a human being. Her age, and her existence are reckoned from her birth...' (cited in Grisez, 1970, p. 360). Thus the fetus became ineligible to recover damages in Tort Law. This view persisted into the late 1930s, when the case of Scott *v.* McPheeters ([1939] Cal. App. 2d 629 cited in Grisez, 1970), in California, allowed that a child '... is deemed to be an existing person from conception provided he is born and survives' (Grisez, 1970, p. 367). It is acknowledged that this case took place in the USA and is cited here for comparative interest but has no legal precedent in the UK. However further cases followed this lead on both sides of the Atlantic and in 1984, in England, a Law Commission Report on Injuries to Unborn Children recommended that: '... the common law would, in appropriate circumstances, provide a remedy for a Plaintiff suffering from a prenatal injury caused by another's fault' (cited in Whitfield, 1993, p. 28).

The Commission endorsed the idea that this recommendation should be supported by legislation. This led to the Congenital Disabilities (Civil Liabilities) Act 1976, which enables a child who is born alive to sue any person, except the mother, who has caused a disability as a result of negligence. Currently the only case where the mother can be sued is if she was driving a car at the time of the alleged incident (Section 2 Congenital Disabilities (Civil Liabilities) Act, 1976).

This, at least, acknowledged a duty of care to the fetus. However he has to be born alive in order to have the capacity to bring an action, and as such the fetus was still not recognized. This was further confirmed in the case of Re F (in utero) (2 F L R: 307 [1988]) where the authorities tried to gain a protection order for the expected child of a nomadic woman whom they considered was putting her fetus at risk. The Court of Appeal confirmed that an unborn child could not be made a ward of court because 'it' has no existence independent of the mother, and they would have to wait until the child was born alive before they could offer protection. However the case of D (a minor) *v.* Berkshire County Council and others ([1987] 1 All ER 20) is worthy of note here because the court was prepared to consider the development and health of the fetus when making their decision. The case involved a local authority attempting to obtain care and control of a child born to a drug addicted mother, claiming that her addiction demonstrated neglect for the child. Again protection was only offered after birth, but it did acknowledge the fetus (Mason and McCall Smith, 1991). Therefore it may be possible for the fetus to gain protection in utero in the future!

The fetus and criminal law

The main focus of attention appears to be in relation to criminal law, in particular to the permissibility or not of abortion throughout the centuries. Archival evidence suggests that there has been an immense variety of social uncertainty about the status of the fetus. It seems to emerge from two sources:

a)   the biological complexities of development, which create discussion about when the fetus becomes a person,
b)   the historical evidence of various moral views on the fetus, which have affected legislation and which vary over time and culture depending on the particular social needs of that era.

Some cultures commonly used abortion and infanticide as methods of controlling fertility (and some continue to do so today (Mosher, 1993), whilst others objected to such acts with differing degrees of severity. Linden (1989) explains that in its earliest stages Roman Law allowed abortion on the grounds that the fetus was only a potential person and still part of its mother. In contrast, some earlier ancient civilizations (Sumerian, Assyrian and Persian cultures) showed some indirect protection towards the fetus by prohibiting the striking of a pregnant woman, as it might damage or cause the death of her fetus.

Early Judaeo-Christian societies condemned abortion by a third party but did not penalize the mother, if she performed it herself. Later this moral and legal focus changed – when the fetus was considered to be a person from the time it was formed (i.e. when it looked like a person). Between the 13th and 17th centuries, it would appear that any punishment by a third party involved in procuring an abortion was left to the ecclesiastical courts, until their decline in the mid seventeenth century following the Reformation (Keown, 1988).

In the 17th century, a noted legal authority, Coke (cited in Linden, 1989) considered that procuring the death of the fetus was not a crime before quickening (when fetal movements can be felt) but it was a serious crime after this event. Keown (1988) writes that with regard to quickening the theory that human life begins at this point originated with Aristotle and was later sustained by Galen. It was also advocated by the Canon Law of the Christian Church and so found its way into common law.

In 1803, Lord Ellenborough's Act provided that all abortion before or after quickening was illegal, but maintained a distinction by having more severe penalties for abortion after quickening. Means (cited in Keown, 1988) contends that the introduction of legislation to outlaw abortion was more to do with preserving maternal, rather than fetal, life. The mortality and morbidity rates for women following attempted abortions was high. This was partly due to ignorance of human biology and widespread use of various 'poisons' administered to induce abortion. The penalty for third party involvement was often a prison sentence. Following the Offences Against the Person Act (1861) women themselves, considered lucky to have survived such dangerous procedures, could have been sentenced to life imprisonment, while the fetus remained incidental to the outcome.

From time to time, a special status has been conferred on the fetus, depending on the severity of the particular legislation governing abortion. For example, in the 18th century, executions of pregnant women were suspended until after the pregnancy was terminated (usually by birth of the child), and later this rule became a permanent stay of execution until in 1931 when the Sentence of Death (Expectant Mothers) Act allowed for a pregnant woman to be given life imprisonment rather than a death sentence (Linden, 1989). It would appear that abortion was not totally prohibited to the point of allowing the mother to die and the case of R *v.* Bourne (1 KB: 689 [1939] cited in Brazier, 1992) established a limited defence of necessity to preserve maternal life. The case involved the prosecution of a doctor for performing a criminal abortion – his defence being that it was to save the mother's life. The case was acquitted when the judge stated that there '... may be a duty to abort to save the "yet more precious" life of the mother' (Brazier, 1992). The term 'life' would appear to have been interpreted broadly, to include both mental and physical well-being and as such this judgement had enabled more women to have easier access to legal abortions. However, the ruling again validated the status of the mother above that of the fetus and suggested that any rights the mother may have supersede those of the fetus.

In 1967, the Abortion Act provided the legal opportunity for women to have abortions. It laid down strict guidelines for when, and by whom, pregnancy termination could be carried out:

STATUTORY GROUNDS AND STATISTICS FOR ENGLAND AND WALES 1992 (OPCS, 1995)

A legally induced abortion, certified by two registered practitioners is justified under one or more of the following statutory grounds:

A the continuance of the pregnancy would involve risk to the life of the pregnant woman greater than if the pregnancy were terminated;

B the termination is necessary to prevent grave permanent injury to the physical or mental health of the pregnant woman;

C the continuance of the pregnancy would involve risk, greater than if the pregnancy were terminated, of injury to the physical or mental health of the pregnant woman;

D the continuance of the pregnancy would involve risk, greater than if the pregnancy were terminated, of injury to the physical or mental health of any existing child(ren) of the family of the pregnant woman;

E there is a substantial risk that if the child were born it would suffer from such physical or mental abnormalities as to be seriously handicapped; *or* in emergency;

F to save the life of the pregnant woman; or

G to prevent grave permanent injury to the physical or mental health of the pregnant woman.

Changes made to the Abortion Act 1967 in 1990 (HF&E Act) included a time limit of 24 weeks for abortions under statutory grounds **C** and **D**. Statutory grounds **A**, **B** and **E** are without a time limit.

In retrospect it would appear that due to the rather liberal interpretation of the Act, it appeared to provide women with an almost unlimited access (in private practice and to a lesser extent on the National Health Service) to legal and safe facilities to terminate an unwanted pregnancy up to 28 weeks gestation and beyond in some specific cases. This was amended in 1990 to 24 weeks, with certain exceptions (HF&E Act, 1990).

There were safeguards built into the 1967 Abortion Act to curb this open availability and once it became apparent that it was not functioning as was intended, several Protection Bills went unsuccessfully before Parliament. However these attempts to provide a more restrictive practice appeared more concerned with the erosion of professional autonomy then with fetal rights, despite some being contested on those grounds (Keown, 1988).

41

The existence of the 1990 (HF&E) Act is viewed by many as a fundamental piece of legislation enabling women to become more autonomous and provide them with an opportunity to control their fertility even further. At the time, and since, numerous debates have challenged women and society about the relative rights of the fetus compared with the apparent total moral rights of the mother to do as she wishes with her body, within the legal framework. Once again it would appear that the fetus had lost out to the mother.

In 1990, the HF&E Act concluded that termination could be conducted up to 24 weeks gestation following heated debate concerning viability. This limit, rather than any of the others proposed, appears to have been chosen because technology has now made it possible for some neonates to survive extra-uterine after 24 weeks gestation. Some unsuccessful attempts were made to reduce this further to 18 weeks. It may be reasonable to suggest that technology has actually improved the legal status of the fetus, by improving his chances of survival.

The father and 'his' fetus: Legal issues

To many the fetus is no longer an undefinable series of cells but a living human being. This may, in part, be related to the use of ultrasound to view the fetus, and such perceptions may have had a positive effect on fathers and society, as well as on mothers (Raphael-Leff, 1991). It may also account for recent moves by some fathers to attempt to gain rights for their unborn children. In 1973, the case of Roe *v*. Wade (93 S Ct 705 (USA) [1973]), in America, confirmed a woman's inalienable prerogative to abortion during the first trimester, despite any objection by a partner or others. In 1978, the case of Paton *v*. British Pregnancy Advisory Service Trustees (QB: 276 [1979] cited in Mason and McCall Smith, 1991) found a husband attempting to 'save' the life of his unborn child when his wife decided to terminate the pregnancy. The judge ruled that the father had no rights, and when it went to the European Commission on Human Rights (arguing the husband's right to family life and the unborn child's right to life), the Commission concluded that the rights of the unborn child were subordinate to the rights of his mother, at least in the initial months of pregnancy. This was further confirmed in the much publicised case of C *v*. S ([1987] All ER:1230), where a partner attempted to stop his ex-girlfriend from terminating her pregnancy. The conclusion again was that it is the woman's right to do with her body (and subsequently any fetus she is carrying) as she chooses.

Embryo research, ownership and the law

The focus of legal attention has now moved towards the New Reproductive Technologies, and discussions about fetal status concern themselves with issues such as:

- embryo research/experimentation and
- ownership of gametes and embryo.

The intention here is to analyse the legal issues surrounding these new developments. Legal attention is concentrating on developments in the area of embryo research because it is likely that any current legal decisions may eventually affect legislation relating to genetic engineering.

Embryo experimentation

(See Chapter 1 for discussion on embryo experimentation)
Over the past century, scientists have been experimenting with animals in attempts to fertilize gametes extra-uterine, but it was not until 1978 that Louise Brown's birth was announced – the first child to have resulted from In Vitro Fertilization (IVF) and successful embryo transfer (Dawson, 1993). Since then, such treatments have become popular worldwide, with a variety of opinions proliferating about the ethics of these therapies and subsequent legal diversity in the laws governing these procedures. In the United Kingdom, the HF&E Act (1990) came into force in 1991, intending to control research into the newly defined pre embryo. Holland (1990) argues that the use of the term pre embryo is intended to deny that human beings begin to exist from conception. The potential value of such a denial may lead to a belief that if the pre embryo is not a person, then experimentation and research carry little or no moral consequences and as such need no protection. In legal terms embryo and pre embryo do appear to be interchangeable at present.

The 1990 Act (HF&E Act) included the statutory licensing of clinical IVF, donation and storage of gametes, and embryo research. After much debate the Act concluded that no research should be conducted beyond 14 days after fertilization. It is believed that the primitive streak appears around 15 days post fertilization, when it becomes possible to identify the developing cell mass as an embryo and as such an individual human being, deserving of some form of protection from inquiring scientists.

The diversity of legislation worldwide reflects the variety of opinions on the personhood of the embryo. Gaze (1990) suggests that it has as much to do with resource allocation as it has to do with the varying consequentialist or deontological views of scientists, parents and society as a whole.

43

There are two main opposing views. On the one hand, scientists and others, opposed to the need for legislation, suggest that they should be left to determine the necessary standards for procedures. They proclaim that they would adapt to public need and would be responsible for the suppression of unacceptable research methods (Walters, 1987). This view would not appear to support any serious notion of the embryo having protection. It also creates concern among those who support a need for formal regulation, suggesting that society may not be prepared to allow the discretion of individual scientists as an adequate 'guarantee' for offering sufficient protection. The problems experienced with Australia's Self Regulation System demonstrates various ethical and practical hazards in sustaining such a system (Kasimba, 1990).

On the other hand, the majority of committees appointed to examine the spectrum of issues surrounding reproductive technologies have found an array of ethical and legal issues which they believe need to be addressed through some form of regulation. In the UK, the Warnock Committee became responsible for the Inquiry into Human Fertilization and Embryology (Warnock, 1985) in 1984. This was later to provide the framework for the HF&E Act in 1990. In asserting the need for regulation of these procedures the report stated that: ' ... the objection to using human embryos in research is that each one is a potential human being. One reference point in the development of the human individual is the formation of the primitive streak' (Warnock, 1985:11.22 p. 66). From this came the recommended 14 day limit on research and prohibition of transferring such embryos to a woman. Once again the embryo has been afforded some protection after it is seen to have some 'human individual status', but not from death (because he can still be legally terminated up to 24 weeks gestation and beyond in some cases!)

The main pro legislation argument is that such research is the 'thin end of the wedge', which could eventually lead to the use of genetic engineering on humans, once the technology has been developed. McLaren (cited in Morgan and Lee, 1991) argued, in 1987, that because it was not possible to replace defective genes with normal ones, this slippery slope view was unrealistic. However, as demonstrated in Chapter 1, the knowledge and understanding of the human genome is progressing daily and supporters believe it is only a matter of time before genetic engineering becomes a human issue (Kelves and Hood, 1993). It should also be noted that even though the Warnock Committee (Warnock, 1985) did not recognize the embryo as a human person, it did state that: 'The status of the human embryo is a matter of fundamental principle which should be enshrined in legislation. We recommend that the embryo of the human species should be afforded some protection in law' (Warnock, 1985: 11.17 p. 63). For future protection, the Human Fertilization and Embryology Authority (HUFEA – the licensing authority set up following the HF&E Act (1990)) have the duty of regularly reviewing developments concerning embryology and human fertilization. The intention is to ensure that the limitations of permissible research are adhered to and, hopefully, to have some control over future developments in this domain.

Ownership of gametes and embryo

Embryo experimentation has also created legal concerns about ownership of gametes and embryo. In order to achieve the research, the necessary gametes need to be available to produce the embryos. Currently they are acquired in two ways:

a)   spare embryos are those created for placement in the woman's uterus, but either because of defect or the woman no longer wants them, they are donated for research;

b)   research embryos are created from anonymously donated eggs and sperm and used exclusively for research.

Worldwide it is generally accepted, but not always enshrined in legislation, that donors have a right to determination prior to donation but after that they have no legal redress with regard to what happens to donated gametes, unless specific instructions were given at the time of donation (Pretorius, 1993).

Donated embryo are stored by a process of cryopreservation, until they are needed for their intended purpose. However, it would appear that the legal concerns only manifest themselves when a problem arises with the prospective parent/s, as demonstrated in the following situations.

In 1984, in Australia, it was revealed that two frozen embryos had been 'orphaned' in 1983, following the unexpected death of their parents (Smith, 1985-86). It was also revealed that donor sperm had been used to fertilize Mrs Rios's eggs. The issues raised were:

1.   did the embryos have a legal right to life, which would have involved finding a surrogate mother for them?

2.   if born alive, would they have any inheritance rights over their parents considerable estate? (Mr and Mrs Rios also had a son from Mr Rios' previous marriage).

It would appear from the literature (Smith, 1985-86) that the case was unresolved as the embryos remained frozen at the medical centre in 1985, by which time they were probably no longer viable anyway (after two years in cryopreservation, the chances of a successful pregnancy are dramatically reduced). However, the case opened discussion on ownership and rights for similar embryos. In August 1984, the Waller Report on the Disposition of Embryos Produced by In Vitro Fertilization concluded that:

> '... the disposition of stored embryo is not to be determined by the hospital where they are stored; that such embryos are not to be regarded as possessing legal rights or having rights to lay claim to inheritance; and in cases where by mischance or for any other reason, an embryo is stored which cannot be transferred as planned, and no agreed provision has been made at the time of storage... the embryos shall be removed from storage.' (Smith, 1985-86, p. 37)

This report was followed by legislation from the Victorian Parliament in Australia (1984) regulating IVF and one of the provisions was that orphaned embryos should be anonymously donated to a woman who could not produce her own eggs (Steinbock, 1992a).

In 1989, in America, the case of Davis *v.* Davis *v.* King M.D. further highlighted the need for appropriate legislation for these unusual circumstances. This case involved a father who was attempting to stop the mother from having their previously frozen embryos being implanted after they had started divorce proceedings (Steinbock, 1992a). (The eggs, aspirated from Mrs Davis in 1981 had been fertilized by Mr Davis' sperm.) Mrs Davis maintained that she was the mother of the embryo's and argued that they had rights of their own. The judge ruled in favour of Mrs Davis, concluding that the embryos were people, not products and based on the 'best interests' analysis it was appropriate that they should be available for implantation. This created controversy about whether embryos were persons or possessions. Judge Young's conclusion suggests that he is an advocate of the 'right to life movement', and opponents of this may well have decided the case differently. Robertson (1989, p. 11), who was among the opponents, considered the conclusion that 'four celled pre implantation human embryos are children and human beings' as unprecedented and unwarranted. The Court of Appeal overturned the decision, awarding *joint control* of the embryos to the Davis's. They made the distinction between joint custody, which would assume the embryos had some legal right to be considered as children, where as joint control does not. The case later went to the Supreme Court (1991) where the appellate decision was largely affirmed (Capon, 1992).

Interestingly, the Supreme Court focused on the 'choices about relationships' and the right to choose *not* to become a parent because 'becoming a parent should involve the freedom to choose, both whether and with whom' (Capon, 1992, p. 32). The court rejected the notion that the embryos were persons in law, particularly because of the existence of abortion laws. They concluded that it was not about the embryos right to life but about Mrs Davis exercising her choice to become a parent over Mr Davis' wishes not to become a parent. It concluded that ideally agreements should be made beforehand as to the future of embryos should one party later decline parenthood, and in this case 'the party wishing to avoid procreation should prevail' (Capon, 1992, p. 33).

Therefore it would appear that the parents should decide beforehand, so avoiding legal proceedings which often leave the embryos in frozen limbo – the longer they wait, the less their chances of survival. Again, parents rights prevail over any rights the embryo might have.

When the HF&E Act 1990 came into being, it attempted to avoid such disputes by stating that ' ... withdrawal of consent of either donor... appears to mean that it must be allowed to perish' (Morgan and Lee, 1991, p. 37). In an attempt to avoid such decision making, the Act (1990) also made it a legal requirement that a will specifying the wishes of both parents with regard to the disposition of the embryos should be made prior to any treatment. However, these guidelines were tested in late 1996 when a Mrs Blood attempted to have infertility treatment using her dead husband's sperm. Unfortunately he was unconscious when the sperm were removed and never gave written consent before his death. HUFEA initially turned down her request to release his sperm on the basis that he did not give written consent, allowing that there is no way of knowing for sure that he would wish to be a father. However, in 1997, Mrs Blood won a final appeal and was given permission by HUFEA to have the sperm exported to another country, where she could attempt to become pregnant.

The 1990s – A time for a change in focus?

The development of gene therapy and understanding of the capacities of the human genome has changed the focus on the fetus from simply life and death. It is no longer a matter of determining whether the fetus has a right to life but a complex set of moral and legal concerns now face those concerned. The law in England does not currently give the fetus any legal status until he is born alive. He is recognized as an entity, whose status deserves some protection but not as a legal person with rights. Brazier (1992) questions this situation especially in relation to how much protection should the fetus be given and at what cost to maternal rights and interests.

Current text does not allow for elaborate discussion about the struggles made by women to develop their rights and ensure that their interests are protected by legal institutions, who could be accused of being male dominated and paternalistic. Suffice to say that women have campaigned vigorously over the years for greater freedom of choice to determine their personal reproductive abilities. Women who choose to have children have lobbied for better conditions and greater autonomy with regard to childbirth, as well as better protection within the work force. For women who choose not to have children, technological developments have enabled them to have greater control over their fertility, and women who need infertility treatment have the assistance of reproductive technologies.

However, it may now be felt by some women that society is moving into an era of 'fetal rights'. Isolated cases of women being involuntarily confined to their bed, ordered to stop taking non prescription drugs and forced to have caesarean sections against their will, for the protection of their fetus, have been filtering through the media from America (Gallagher, 1986). This has led to some states, including Georgia and California, creating legal statutes that equate the 'criminally caused death of a fetus with murder', if it can be proved that the death was caused by fetal abuse. Field (1989) argues that the current movement towards this concern for maintaining a safe environment for the fetus may not necessarily be in danger of overturning the rights women have acquired, but they may, if taken far enough, curtail and control their behaviour during pregnancy. She elaborates on a movement in America, interested in protecting the fetus and child where '... advocates have called for legislatures to prescribe the conduct of pregnant women, for District Attorneys to prosecute women who "abuse their fetus", and for the state to remove the child at birth' (Field, 1989, p. 114).

Does the development of such movements suggest that the fetus may gain some legal power of protection from his mother (or parents) in the future? And how could such a law be enforced? There appears to be a sense of the previously quoted observation by Gentles (1990) (Chapter 1) whereby the fetus could have the power to be protected from abuse but not from the ultimate abuse of death! This point will be returned to later, but it is worthy of note that the Congenital Disabilities (Civil Liabilities) Act 1976 only excluded the mother from negligence if she was driving a car, and so excludes the child from bringing a claim for negligence as a result of alcohol or drug abuse, unless she was involved in a car accident at the time of injury!

In 1991 the case of Re S (All E R 4:671 [1992]) demonstrated, for the first time in English legal history, the power of the fetus at birth in comparison to the mother's right (Morgan, 1992). In this case the mother refused to consent, on religious grounds, to have a caesarean section despite being aware of the possible risks to herself and her fetus. The Health Authority went to court to obtain permission to 'save' her and her baby, this was granted and despite her objections the operation went ahead – unfortunately the child did not survive the ordeal. Under current legislation a woman has the legal right to do as she wishes with her fetus (for example, she can terminate her pregnancy, with considerable risk to the fetus up to 24 weeks and sometimes beyond that limit) yet when it came to her autonomous decision with regard to her body and her viable fetus she was overruled – the justification for this being the life of her unborn child – someone who has no legal status. Steinbock (1992b) remarks that such coercive behaviour from the professionals is aimed at protecting the future child, not the fetus. It is also possible that such decisions may have more to do with personal moral beliefs, about the rights of the viable fetus, being imposed in a paternalistic way. In England this is an isolated case (In 1996 another case of 'forced caesarean section' made the headlines. However the mental competance of the mother, due to schizophrenic illness, was the cause for concern and, although it caused outrage, was viewed differently – see Tameside and Glossop Acute Services Trust *v.* CH [1996] 1 FLR) for details). Notwithstanding this, cases have been documented elsewhere, and although they have no legal precedence in UK law, are worthy of note in the light of future possibilities. Kluge (1988) reviews a variety of similar cases in Canada and argues that one should be willing to balance the rights of the mother with that of the fetus. However he concludes that when cases come to court the fetus usually wins! There is a strong suspicion that moral thinking is informing legal judgements – killing innocents is not morally justifiable, which is presumably how these mothers who refuse treatment at the cost to their fetus, are viewed.

At present the law is largely reactive rather than proactive – choosing to build case law rather than enact legislation on fetal rights. One concern is that these decisions are usually taken following a short deliberation, due to the nature of the situation, the case of Re S being decided in less than half an hour. However concerns that it may stand as precedent for future cases has largely been rejected, especially in the light of the Royal College of Obstetricians and Gynaecologists Report (RCOG, 1994, Para 5.12, p. 15) recommending that in future such operations should not be performed, when the woman refuses to consent to treatment. Nevertheless that does not necessarily mean that the fetus will not attain some protection in the future – the public may well call for a more balanced view in the 'rights' of the mother versus the rights' of the fetus debate.

Conclusion

In legal terms, the status of the fetus and embryo appears to vary depending on the particular issues at stake. Regardless of debates about who should have priority, mother or fetus, the fact remains that they are inseparable and so a balance has to be struck. The father, as we have seen, has no rights of determination about 'his' fetus.

Historically the fetus was seen more as a vehicle for obtaining rights and seems to have some indirect protection for this purpose. Looking at property rights, cases involving unborn children were more to do with maintenance of titles and ownership of property. In tort law, protection was provided so that *if* the child survived he may have some redress for injury, *if* negligence is proved.

Criminal law, concerned with abortion, has developed around benefits to the mother, and supporters of the fetus appear to come second place. In contrast to that today, attempts to control the mother's freedom during pregnancy may be seen as a move towards greater tolerance and understanding of the need for fetal status. However the practical issues of enforcing such ideals still remain problematic.

In the past decade, the focus has been on the less recognizable fetus, the embryo and/or pre embryo, and it would appear that the pre embryo has lost any possibility of 'human status' being bestowed, following successive legislation allowing 'experimentation' and 'disposal' up to 14 days gestation. The evolution of the human genome adds to the dilemmas facing society, especially as the advantages envisaged appear to be beneficial to many.

However, concern still remains. If we do not treat the embryo/pre embryo with some respect (and subsequent legal protection), are we in danger of creating more problems than we can imagine for the future? Or will regulation and 'good sense' prevail to provide reasoned and scientifically balanced discussion to resolve potential problems?

Meyers (1990) argues that the law cannot wait and watch, that it should develop a legally sound and socially acceptable rationale for dealing with these conflicts. The time has passed for assuming that, in all cases, the mother's rights will prevail over all else, the fetus has gained some recognition in recent years and the trend appears to be continuing, especially in relation to the age of viability. However the pre embryo would appear to be viewed as pre individual human being undeserving of protection or special status and may provide opportunities for human genetic engineering in the future.

CHAPTER FOUR

The Future: Moral and Legal Justification and Control

Introduction

Genes have two vital functions, they carry our inheritance package and are responsible for numerous aspects of protein production – they are responsible for keeping human beings alive. They have been regarded as very complex molecules and until recently, understanding of their specific functions and sequencing has been limited. Now that HUGO is producing information, almost daily, the future of genetics is looking rather different to a decade or two ago. It is largely assumed that further research will lead to more genetic testing/profiling, prenatal diagnosis (and even pre conception prediction) of genetic disease, human gene therapy and research into the pre disposition of various disease states (Pompidou, 1995).

It has been hailed as a new and exciting age of discovery, unprecedented in history, yet many authors temper their excitement with cautionary tales of concern about how far these disclosures will take the human race. Will it be just about understanding ourselves better with a focus on individual disease states and attempting to cure/eliminate such illnesses as Huntington's Chorea, Cystic Fibrosis and some cancers, or are we embarking on a new age of eugenics? Will eugenic treatments be viewed positively or negatively, and how far will society go towards producing perfect human beings – and who will define the criteria for these perfect persons? This also raises questions about the effects to individual or collective moral views about any special status for the embryo including how any changes may affect legislation.

The previous two chapters demonstrated that living in a pluralistic society reflects different views, depending on one's belief about when any special or personhood status should be bestowed. Legally the embryo can be experimented on and discarded up to 14 days gestation, then protected from such research after that, yet he can have his life terminated up to 24 weeks gestation (and beyond in some specific cases). However, if he survives the fetal and birthing processes, and is born with a disability resulting from negligence, he then has a legal personality, and as such can bring a claim for negligence under the Congenital Disabilities (Civil Liabilities) Act 1976.

Why is birth such a great divider? Is it, as Glover (1990) suggests, merely related to a sentimentality of seeing a helpless newborn with a 'personality' of his own? If a woman had a transparent uterus, would our sentimental views recede to sometime during the gestation? Perhaps such a question is unanswerable. However setting boundaries either at viability, birth or beyond has major implications for the embryo and fetus. The value of these boundaries lie in their usefulness in justifying research on, or death to, a developing human being who cannot object to his life being interfered with or terminated.

On account of the widespread disagreement about the status of the fetus and embryo, perhaps the question posed should focus more on whether *the Human Genome Knowledge Explosion will affect our thinking about the various theories behind the development of personhood and what impact these changes may have on current legislation,* rather than on what effects the new knowledge may have on the legal and moral status of the fetus and embryo.

With this change of thought in mind, the central question remains, but the focus may be more varied, based on the idea that there is no single status. This chapter will concentrate firstly on the specific ethical issues relating to the moral status of the embryo and fetus following the revelations about the human genome. Secondly, from a legal perspective, attention will be focused on the legal problems which may arise. The whole issue of ownership and patentability of the knowledge discovered is relevant to the future of the embryo and this will include discussion about the commercial value of this information. One apprehension is that a 'commercial value' attitude may force a change in moral thinking about the status of the embryo, and if this is so, will it create changes in the law? This will also lead to a consideration of potential regulation and control of these practices.

As this is a new and futuristic subject, some speculation is necessary, based on current knowledge.

The embryo, the fetus and the future

The use of the knowledge produced by the Human Genome initiative is vast, and appears to have the potential to alter the abilities of science and medicine in the future. Genetic engineering is a fact and it raises many ethical and legal concerns, not least in relation to the embryo and fetus. Any genetic therapies to be used may begin the road of success or failure with embryo experimentation, therefore consideration has to be given to the effects of these developments on the embryo and fetus.

Before considering what can be done, some discussion is necessary in relation to the topic of genetic selection – is it really necessary and good? It would appear that the answer is yes, especially if one considers the extent of interest and resources which have been used in developing the knowledge and techniques. There are, however, concerns and anxieties which cannot be ignored. The concept of genetic selection does need serious consideration, especially if future issues of discrimination and failure are to be minimized. Should society consider altering the genetic makeup of individuals or sections of society? For those who suffer from debilitating genetic disease then it would appear immoral to withhold helpful treatments.

However, the problem is then deciding what is debilitating or serious. The concept of defining 'normal' and 'abnormal' appear to have little consensus. Nevertheless to accept that genetic manipulation is morally permissible for some and not for others, based on some form of social criteria, could be considered discriminatory.

Various authors (Greely, 1993; Nelkin, 1993; Harris, 1993; Watt, 1993) are expressing concern about specific aspects of potential discrimination in education, employment, health and insurance issues for those who may be genetically susceptible to diseases or 'undesirable' traits. For example, Skene (1991) reported on a genetic screening project in Greece, where carriers of the sickle cell gene were stigmatized by a community and considered ineligible for marriage. Also, in February 1997, the Association of British Insurers produced an information leaflet (related to a policy statement on Life Insurance and Genetics), which clearly suggests that such organizations would expect to use all possible information available (including genetic profiling) to make accurate assessments of risks. The concern here would be how significant possible predicted risks in adulthood, or risks for the women who may reproduce a child with genetic abnormalities, may influence ability to acquire life insurance etc. Is this just the tip of the new genetic 'iceberg'?

As the majority of these issues concern children and adults they will not be pursued in depth here. However it is necessary to draw attention to them, as awareness by parents of such potential problems may influence their decisions in relation to their embryo.

HUGO is an information gathering project and genetic engineers have to effectively use the information gained for successful manipulation, which will inevitably create a gap between knowledge and technology. Subsequently, the short term effects on the embryo and fetus could be devastating. It is possible that prenatal diagnostic tests will increase but with no treatment or positive prognosis, the only options for parents may be to continue with the pregnancy and hope for developments, or terminate the pregnancy. Current practice suggests that the latter would appear to be favoured by many with high expectations for normal children.

This issue of parental and social expectation of normality may have a major influence on what may or may not be allowed in the future. Why do these expectations exist, especially within such pluralist societies? Is it associated with a social and personal pressure/human need to 'fit-in' and not be different? Or is it 'easier' to bring up 'normal' children, to enable parent's to continue with career patterns or other interests? Should society take a more serious view of the adjustments that parents have to make, or should be prepared to make, when they take on the responsibility of children? Is it resource driven? Children and adults with physical disabilities need special equipment, buildings adapted to meet their needs and possibly more medical treatment. Those with learning disabilities have different (possibly more expensive) care, educational and employment needs. If they become an even smaller minority than present, will their rights be marginalized as well?

The reasons for this perceived need for 'normal, healthy' children are probably multi-factorial but does appear to be an increasing expectation of society, which may put the embryo and fetus at further risk of manipulation in the future.

Another concern could take the form of increased embryo research to develop treatments or test hypotheses about gene/gene sequence activity. The potential benefits from embryo research and tissue transplantation appear enormous (see Chapter 1) and the implied good that could be derived for a variety of people cannot be overlooked. However the question still remains – will genetic engineering change individual and collective beliefs about the moral status of the embryo and fetus?

For those who believe that the embryo does not have any right to personhood status until he is viable or born or knows what it is to have a right, then this issue may pose few ethical dilemmas because the embryo will probably be viewed as a form of raw material to be enhanced, thereby producing a better person later. Of course this view is not categorical and some may still object to genetic manipulation on the grounds of slippery slope arguments or the issue of altering the identity of what the cells may become.

Another issue that has to be considered is that of using embryos for the enhancement of others. In Chapter 1, speculation occurred about the possibility of building a 'cloned embryo store' for spare parts which could be used as material to be grafted to a 'better' (more developmentally advanced) human being. Although it is somewhat futuristic, it deserves mention here because of the principle involved in using one 'human being' for another's benefit, and it is an issue for the embryo because he cannot consent to or object to his body being used to benefit someone else, possibly to the total detriment of his own.

The nearest society has come to this at present was demonstrated in a news report entitled 'When One Body Can Save Another' (Morrow, 1991). It relayed the story of a mother who deliberately conceived a child in the hope that he/she would provide essential bone marrow to be transplanted to an older sick sibling. The marrow transplant presented few risks for the new child, provided he/she survived the fetal and birthing process, but the case created a great deal of controversy. Zucker (1992) states that public outcry from ethicists was largely negative but a survey conducted by the magazine suggested that 47 per cent of respondents considered it 'morally acceptable for parents to conceive a child in order to obtain an organ or tissue to save the life of another', whereas 37 per cent disagreed. (The survey did not specify how many, or what section of the population, took part, which could have significance with regard to the result.) It could be argued that a child was created that would not have been otherwise, and as discussed earlier, it is better to have existed than not, but what of the scenario when embryo may be created and stored, only for their organs, and not for any chance of life?

From a conservative viewpoint the position is categorical, the embryo and fetus deserve to be treated with respect and have moral rights from conception. Any manipulation of an embryo for research and information gathering is unacceptable and disrespectful to the embryo. However, if such therapies were to benefit that person in later life, would it be morally wrong not to do all one could to enhance their life prospects? Conservative thinkers would have to question whether the means justified the ends. The 'means' would, by the nature of the work being conducted, have involved earlier experimentation on some embryos to develop and verify the safety and success of the therapies!

An example of how this may work in practice was demonstrated recently with the measles and rubella campaign. In 1994, when the government announced a mass vaccination campaign, the headmaster of Ampleforth Catholic Boys School 'forbade' the vaccine in his school on the grounds that his pupils should not benefit from an 'evil act' (Kenny, 1994). The evil act he was referring to was that the vaccine being used had originated (in 1966) from material derived from an aborted fetus (Mihill and Ward, 1994). It is acknowledged that although this fetus was already dead when experimented on, the principle of respect for the human fetus, and use of one solely for someone else's benefit remains the same.

Such a pronouncement had potentially serious consequences for Catholic parents and their children. The media followed this original story with another, the headline ran 'Vaccination urged by Catholics' (Mihill and Ward, 1994), reporting that many Catholic parents were urging others to ensure that their children were vaccinated because of the potential devastating effects of the illnesses. In February 1995, there was a follow-up report by Mihill (1995) which declared the campaign a success, with the lowest number of cases reported in January.

When it comes to individual choice, it is reasonable to see that parents will do anything within their power to protect and enhance the life of their child/ren. Even if collectively, people who would be seen to follow conservative beliefs, and may feel uncomfortable or negative towards embryo research, will naturally choose what is seen to be most beneficial for their family. Does this then suggest that the means may justify the ends, and if people begin to focus on 'what would I do if it was my personal decision...' it may be possible to justify developments in genetic engineering at the expense of some embryos?

Will genetic engineering change collective or individual views on the moral status of the embryo and fetus?

The developments in genetics have altered our understanding of the fetus and embryo. Firstly, knowledge of the activities of genes and gene sequencing has led to greater understanding of our capacities and limitations. Secondly, it has led to major advances in treating genetic disease and genetic engineering techniques. Thirdly, it has led to advances in science and medicine for children and adults, some of which have been initiated using the embryo.

There are numerous other developments, which will not be elaborated on here, apart from the concept of the pre embryo (Holland, 1990). It would appear that debate about the opportunities for the future has allowed the early developing embryo to be referred to in terminology that suggests he is something less than that (Jones and Telfer, 1995), and this has significance when considering the positive and negative aspects of such research. It must be reiterated again that any practices used on the pre embryo, the embryo or the fetus appear directly related to the notion of when personhood develops. Chapter 2 provided extensive analysis of this issue and the conclusion was that of two very diverse sets of values and beliefs. There are those who believe that the embryo (from conception) is a human entity and because of this potential to become a thinking moral person, he should be afforded protection and respect that reflects that position. In direct opposition there are those who, for a variety of reasons, believe that personhood and human development do not begin at the same time and therefore it is possible to justify experimentation on the early embryo because 'it' is not a person and so cannot be harmed by anything done to 'it'.

To determine the moral effects on the fetus and embryo certain questions (see Fig. 4.1) have to be considered in relation to morally justifying particular aspects of the proposals.

Is it morally justifiable to:

1. Genetically select future human beings?
2. Create embryos for research?
3. Use these embryos in experimentation?
4. Use embryo for the possible benefit of others?
5. Genetically manipulate the embryo:
   i) to correct a genetic defect?
   ii) to enhance a genetic defect?
   iii) to alter the gene pool?
6. Diagnose disease when no treatment or preventative measures are available?
7. Potentially increase the number of therapeutic abortions, until effective treatments or preventative measures are available?
8. Use genetic engineering techniques on human beings with known and unknown consequences?

Fig. 4.1

1. Is it morally justifiable to genetically select future human beings?
The whole issue of genetic selection appears to have been taken for granted (in some circles) as being a positive move. However we live in a world of limited resources, and consideration should be made with regard to the use of these resources. Could they be put to better use in helping those who are disabled and in attempting to find alternative treatments, rather than using embryos to experiment on? The current route proposed may produce more 'perfect' people but there is a real danger that this will only add to the current discrimination towards those seen to be disabled, either from genetic fault or accident (e.g. road traffic or sports injuries).

The other issue in relation to genetic selection is that of failure. It would not appear possible to give guarantees of success and so preparation would have to be made for dealing with unsuccessful genetic manipulation, where the desired effect was not achieved or the genes spontaneously mutated creating undesired effects. Is this worth the risk to the embryo, who may end up being terminated if all is not well?

2. Is it morally justifiable to create embryos for research?

3. Is it morally justifiable to use these embryos in experimentation?

4. Is it morally justifiable to use embryos for the possible benefit of others?

There are major concerns with creating and using embryos just as a means to an end. Utilitarian views justify it as absolutely necessary, and the benefits seem to far outweigh the 'sacrifice' of some embryos. However, in recalling the conservative viewpoint the embryo deserves respect and if such a consensus is to be maintained then there has to be consideration of the real need for this research. It may be possible to focus research on gametes before fertilization or even on adults with their consent. It would suggest that because legislation has allowed embryo research, there appears to be few resources being used in search of acceptable alternatives. One such alternative is the Life Hospital Trust, based in Liverpool. It is a pro life organization focusing on issues such as infertility and natural family planning, who are in the process of developing a research centre that will not involve embryo research.

Another area of concern is that there appears to be little explicit information about the number of embryos who have been destroyed following research (explicit data is available on abortions carried out), which again suggests that these pre embryo do not even deserve recognition for the contributions they are making to this 'essential' research. The HUFEA do not keep statistics on the numbers of embryos used in research. They expect each centre involved to submit data (on application for research licence renewal) on the number of embryos expected to be used, and at the end of the year (licences are only issued annually) data on the numbers actually used. This does rely somewhat on the integrity of individuals, with any major discrepancy between the two being investigated by HUFEA (Heales, 1995, personal communication). However there is no central statistical information collated, and if such information was needed, inquiries would have to be made to each centre involved in research.

The numerous justifications for embryo research apparently validate the continuance of this work. However if protection of the fetus and embryo are to be considered seriously then attention has to be focused on other means of gaining this knowledge – we live in the computer age where simulations bring interactive programmes which can be altered and developed. Is it possible to consider this as an option for those working in this field? Perhaps more national and international co-operation and exchange of ideas would enable a change of direction which would benefit the presently disadvantaged embryo?

5. Is it morally justifiable to genetically manipulate the embryo:
   i) to correct a genetic defect?
   ii) to enhance a genetic defect?
   iii) to alter the gene pool?

If genetic selection and embryo research is justifiable, then manipulation is part of the same process in terms of ethical concerns. The importance for the embryo would appear to be how far these therapies will go. It seems reasonable to speculate that correction of genetic faults will be the first priority, but again how will genetic defect be defined? Consider the scenario of an embryo who has a predicted adult height of 4' 10", with parent/s who aspire to having tall children because they believe (or society expects) tall people to succeed better! It would be possible to argue that this embryo is 'defective' and such a social expectation could be paralleled with the *expectation* today of 'normal' people having two functional arms and legs. This expectation is evident today in the need to 'encourage' (sometimes by legislation) the adaptation of equipment and buildings for people who do not meet *current social expectations* on physical normality. The line between corrective enhancement and eugenic therapies is thin and it would appear that if the technology is available then not using it would be difficult to justify. Such scenarios have little consideration for the embryo, who is viewed as 'potentially defective and in need of fixing' before being allowed to develop.

6. Is it morally justifiable to diagnose disease when no treatment or preventative measures are available?

7. Is it morally justifiable to potentially increase the number of therapeutic abortions, until effective treatments or preventative measures are available?

There is an entire ethical debate regarding the issue of diagnosing disease when no treatment or preventative measures are available, which will not be elaborated on here. However the concerns for the fetus, as well as the many pre implanted embryos consigned to the waste disposal unit or wherever, has to be raised. The number of embryos who may perish during experimentation is potentially phenomenal, especially as explicit information is not available, in particular in this country, which has a regulation body. What about countries who have less rigorous controls? This would not include the increased risk of spontaneous abortion following genetic manipulation if it was unsuccessful. It must be remembered that once in vitro genetic manipulation is completed, the embryo has to be returned to the uterus, and the success rates of this process remain low (HUFEA, 1995). It would also appear that such practices are liable to increase the number of therapeutic abortions as parents seek normality for their children and prospective adults. Such an increase in therapeutic abortions would do little to improve the status of the fetus if such practices gained further 'popularity', as a means to an end. One author (Kevles and

Hood, 1992) refers to a case where a woman with two sons, equally at risk of developing Huntington's Chorea, requested a genetic test on both in order to determine which will get the better education as she could not afford to send both to university! What if this profile could be done on the embryo – would termination be the option for parents in this or similar situations?

To those who believe in the rights of the embryo and fetus, it may seem indefensible to create and then destroy a fetus who has an incurable disease or undesirable trait, but it must be remembered that this is what happens at present with genetic disorders – for those diagnosed with Down's Syndrome, for example, the only *cure* may be to terminate the pregnancy! It is acknowledged that parents do not deliberately create a fetus with genetic disorders, the intention here is to question the right of parent/s to destroy the fetus because he has a genetic disorder.

Perhaps society should attempt to engender a greater sense of reproductive responsibility with improved pre conception care and perhaps pre pregnancy profiles to assess risk ratios. A greater onus should also be placed on planning a family with more contraceptive choice and support. Again the issue of public debate and accurate information must be to the fore to enable responsible decision making.

8. Is it morally justifiable to use genetic engineering techniques on human beings with known and unknown consequences?

Caution must be exercised if these procedures are to be carried out. It has been emphasized again that a great deal of research is needed to ensure safety and positive results. If germ line cell therapy is to be considered, careful deliberation is necessary, not just for current practice but also for future possibilities.

Even with such careful consideration, there are potential 'unknowns' that cannot even be speculated about at this time, and for this reason it may be justifiable to challenge the need for genetic manipulation of the human embryo. The absolute negative prospect could be the potential to destroy the human race, or significant parts of it – is this possible or simply science fiction at its worst? Harris reminds us that, 'We should not forgo the benefits for fear that we will not have the courage to outlaw the harms' (Harris, 1993, p. 218). Notwithstanding that, it has to be remembered that by their very nature, genes and Recombinant DNA have an unpredictability that cannot currently be harnessed, so outlawing the practice when the damage is done may be too late.

All of the above and numerous other ethical issues will create diverse conversation presently and in the future. The overall benefits are vast (Glover et al., 1989) but it would not appear to bode well for the embryo and fetus. It seems that as practices become more acceptable, safer and better, the greater their use will be. As demonstrated with the measles vaccine, it would appear reasonable to expect parents to do whatever they can for their particular children and make use of the resources available to them, despite any 'shady' past (concerning other embryos) that may have made it possible.

On the other hand, an attempt to outlaw embryo experimentation now may be necessary if the embryo is to be protected. As stated earlier, resources could be increased to consider other viable options. If this is considered realistically then there may be some hope of gaining a greater status in the future. Such an option may depend on whether a majority vote would work towards the embryo being considered a potential person with humanistic characteristics or a 4–8 celled pre embryo of raw material to be moulded to meet future demands.

Ward (1990) acknowledged that some ethical issues are irresolvable, but that does not exclude them from discussion. Rational debate should be based on a fully informed analysis of the facts, which may lead to a 'common commitment to achieve a coherent and defensible overall ethical view' (Ward, 1990, p. 119). However, it is difficult to imagine how such reasoned debate will lead to a situation which encompasses all positions on the moral status of the embryo.

Genetic material and commercial value: is it intellectual property?

There is a concern that genetic engineering practices may be pursued because of the potential economic benefits and these issues cannot be overlooked when considering the effects on the fetus. Subsequently it becomes necessary to focus on ownership, rights of access and the commercial value of the knowledge (see Fig. 4.2).

This new knowledge can be divided into:

a) explanation of genes and the significance of their relationship to other genes/gene sequences, towards a greater understanding of inherited traits;

b) use of this information in genetic engineering, and its application to plants, animals and human beings.

Fig. 4.2

It is noteworthy that the significant issue relating to ownership is in the unique ability of genes to carry *human* genetic information (Jansen, 1985). As with any new 'invention', genetic engineering has significant commercial value, in terms of research developments, product manufacture and sales. Booth (1992) suggests that some 20 per cent of total costs in industry go in research developments, which explain why any science based industry would want some return on their investment, including protection of any new discoveries. In the case of genetic engineering, the new discoveries often relate to human genetic material, and this raises concern because of the possibility of owning part of a human being.

In legal terms, issues of ownership and access to information draw attention to *confidentiality* and *intellectual property law*. The latter is described by Phillips and Firth as the '... rights which are enjoyed in the province of the mind, rather than upon the product itself' (1990, p. 3). Hoffman and Karny suggested that intellectual property is becoming increasingly important in terms of assets, '... it is the vehicle by which society nurtures the creative efforts of its people, recognizes those efforts and protects their fruits from misappropriation' (1988, p. 359). If the information gained from biotechnological methods is considered intellectual property, and there is some debate about this, then the question of ownership may become of international importance.

Intellectual property is a concept rather than a material or product, therefore in terms of genetic engineering, one is concerned with the issues of who owns, and who should have access to, any developments. Patenting does appear to be more important than just copyrights because companies could claim a licence fee if someone used the results of their work, whereas if it was copyrighted, a payment is only due on its reproduction, not its application (Booth, 1992).

Confidentiality about methods used and information gained raises immense legal concerns, especially in relation to how far legislation may be prepared to go to protect such information. Brahams reminds us that British law, which does protect against a breach of confidentiality, is basically reactive and therefore any problems posed by '... futuristic medico-scientific discoveries are likely to be dealt with by reference to established legal principles and analogies made with decided cases' (1990, p. 111). One could argue that, due to the unprecedented nature of the knowledge being developed, such activities may prove difficult.

Brahams (1990) explains that in an attempt to 'protect' the knowledge behind 'DNA fingerprinting' or 'profiling', a company, ICI Diagnostics (in agreement with the Lister Institute of Preventive Medicine and Professor Alex Jeffreys, who discovered the process in 1984) have applied for international patents and have been granted a British patent for the processes involved. The success of biotechnological methods (e.g. DNA fingerprinting) achieving a patent may lead to opportunities for other genetically engineered techniques having access to patent law, including those involving plants and animals. The aim of patent law is to stimulate technological advancement and the general perception was that plants and animals are 'products of nature' and therefore are not patentable (and subsequent arguments could be reasonably applied to include human beings) (Hoffman and Karny, 1988). However the idea of excluding plant and animal patents would appear to be changing, with patents being granted for micro-organisms and genetically engineered organisms. In 1988, in the USA, a patent was issued for the 'Harvard Mouse' which was genetically engineered (Blair and Rowan, 1990). However Phillips and Firth (1990) reported that the European Patent Office refused the patent application for this transgenic animal in 1990. 'Transgenic' is the term used to describe plants and animals which have been altered as a result of genetic engineering.

The issue of patenting information about the human genome will create even greater concern. The notion of owning a part of the 'human being' does not appear acceptable. Perhaps it is reminiscent of slavery and other historical events, now considered to be politically incorrect, which focused on the 'right' of one individual to 'own' another! It may also become necessary to consider just what should be patented, for example the technology behind the Recombinant DNA techniques or the knowledge of the gene sequencing, or both? Mellor (1988) suggests that because cloning techniques have been developed to such an extent that knowledge of the DNA sequence is not a prerequisite to obtaining a clone, therefore a patent for protection may already be redundant!

Booth (1992) contends that there are practical issues with patenting a gene or gene sequence because it is a description of something that already exists and as such it is not an invention! A further problem lies with the scientist who may try to patent a gene sequence. One of the criteria for patenting is that the invention must be useful; by the very nature of the HUGO project, gene sequencing does not fulfil that criteria when discovered, and by the time utility can be demonstrated, the product (i.e. the gene/gene sequence) would no longer be new. In the USA and Japan this problem has been overcome by introducing a period of grace during which disclosure of information would not prejudice a subsequent application for a patent (Booth, 1992). At present the legislation in the UK is ambiguous and it is difficult to predict whether the Patent Office would accept an application to patent part of the human genome. However there is concern that the commercial value and viability of science based industries may prevail over moral concerns about this issue of patenting. This point also raises concerns about removing valuable information from the public domain (Brahams, 1990). This was further confirmed, in July 1997, in discussions leading up to the European Parliaments approval of a European

Union Directive allowing pharmaceutical firms to patent genes. This was in support of progress on genetic research into plants and animals, and reassurance was given that genetic research using human cloning remains prohibited at present (Palmer, 1997).

The question to be answered by the legal system is, whether human genetic material can be considered as intellectual property and deserving of some legal protection, possibly in the form of a patent? Or whether it is significant to public interest and as such should be freely and easily available? Pompidou argues for a balance whereby the human genome is protected from ownership on the basis that '... no one can have the right to monopolise a discovery, as every discovery is part of the natural order to which human beings themselves belong' (1995, p. 70). He also states that there should be some form of fair reward, either financial gain or social recognition, for the processes involved something akin to the legal protection of software.

There are other issues relating to long term economic viability and questions relating to resource allocation for such therapies. When available, will they be offered openly or selectively? Silverman (1995) considers the 'marketplace' influences that may operate in these developments and speculates that some costs may be passed down to unsuspecting parents, which could have a major influence on availability.

It would appear that patenting and ownership of these techniques may not directly influence the embryo. However there may be indirect effects based on the commercial viability of these technologies – after all utility of the 'product' may have to be verified using research embryos for proof of their usefulness. Another indirect problem could be that if techniques are patented and access is restricted, further embryo research may be considered necessary to develop other cheaper techniques. It would also appear that regulation and laws governing ownership and use of information gained should, as always, take account of social and ethical needs as well as commercial expectations and desires. However only the future will demonstrate which will take precedent.

Control and regulation

There appears to be an assumption that genetic engineering techniques for human beings will happen, as the potential benefits are immense and the HF&E Act (1990), in its current form, may not legally cover all eventualities. As discussed earlier, many interested parties believe that there is a legitimate need for regulation, especially as it will involve human beings. The nature of the diversity of opinions and anxieties about these therapies suggest the need for a multidisciplinary group that could fairly represent a pluralistic society.

Opportunity will need to be provided for extensive and frank debate about how far these therapies can realistically work – will they just be about the use of corrective therapies or will it be possible and acceptable to contemplate and justify the use of germ line eugenic practices? The issue of public debate is important for acceptance of these therapies as well as realistic understanding of their limits and uses. Dixon (1993) reminds readers that lack of public consultation before the use of genetically engineered foodstuffs has created more anxiety about the realities of the technology. He suggests that the government took a rather paternalistic view of a public 'need to know', which may have led to greater suspicion about these products.

This implies that public awareness and understanding is significant, and regulation by a responsible body may help to alleviate the specific concerns that these therapies raise. In order to demonstrate their legitimacy, this group would have to hold respect and some power to regulate and manage new developments – who should be responsible? Skene (1991) suggests a template for possible regulation (see Fig. 4.3).

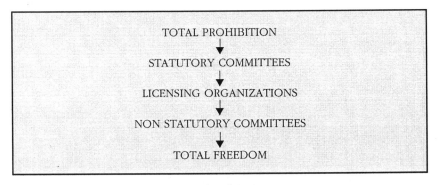

TOTAL PROHIBITION

STATUTORY COMMITTEES

LICENSING ORGANIZATIONS

NON STATUTORY COMMITTEES

TOTAL FREEDOM

Fig. 4.3

Each option can provide various degrees of control. The idea of society placing total prohibition on all activities may be attractive to those who believe in the special status or potential personhood of the embryo from conception. However it seems unlikely that the HF&E Act (1990) will be abolished at this stage, especially as there is quite an impressive list of potential benefits.

The other end of the spectrum is total freedom for scientists, and this would appear equally unacceptable, especially in the light of concerns about possible manipulative eugenic practices and discrimination towards or against those who have had genetic engineering therapies.

The alternatives left fall between the two extremes and Skene (1991) describes three of these:

1.   A Statutory Committee, which would be responsible for approving any activities, with a legal power of imposing some form of criminal sanction if rules or guidelines were not adhered to;
2.   A Licensing Authority, which would have more of a civil right of action rather than criminal basis for imposing its control;
3.   A Non Statutory Committee, consisting mostly of scientists with other appropriate representatives. Such a group may have the power to dictate standards but would have little authority to impose them.

Embryo research is currently regulated by the HUFEA and John Hannan MP summarized the need for such legislation thus '... legislation was necessary to regulate research on embryos, to protect the integrity of reproductive medicine, and to protect scientists and clinicians from legal actions and sanctions' (Morgan and Lee, 1991, p. 22). Interestingly, it says little about protecting the embryo and more about protection of the professional involved. Currently the HUFEA focuses on inspection and licensing of centres involved in donor insemination treatment, IVF and embryo research. The Annual Report for 1992–93 (HUFEA 1994, p. 2) states that the members '... ensure that human embryos are used responsibly and that infertile patients are not exploited at a vulnerable time'.

The membership of the authority professes to be broad, with at least 50 per cent not involved in health care or scientific practices (they include law, religion, finance and the media). However it is noteworthy that an attempt to ensure a balance of people in favour of and opposed to embryo research was defeated when the act was being established. Morgan and Lee (1991) suggest that such a proposal was considered a 'wrecking amendment' as the purpose of the authority was to research the embryo!

This does somewhat suggest a certain need for self regulation with actual practices, and does not necessarily put forward a balanced view for society as a whole. A glance at the actual membership may further confirm this lack of balance, which was perhaps intentional, after all the primary purpose suggests that embryo experimentation is acceptable, provided it is regulated!

It is equally reasonable to propose that because of the unprecedented nature of genetic engineering, a more balanced view is essential and as such a different type of regulating body (either to work with or replace HUFEA) may be necessary.

New legislation may also be necessary in relation to actual embryo research (if it is to continue). If (when) genetic engineering becomes available for human embryos, it would appear necessary to allow for genetic manipulation and subsequent implantation of the embryo for growth and development. HF&E Act Section 3(3)(a) 1990 does not currently allow embryo used in experimentation to be implanted. This will inevitably lead to renewed and extended debates about the wisdom of progress in the use and abuse of these embryo.

Conclusion

The Human Genome Project and subsequent genetic engineering techniques promise significant changes in the way inherited diseases and traits will be managed in the future. The overriding issue in protecting future generations would appear to be the need for adequate regulation and control of any developments. This must be accompanied by appropriate, extensive and honest public debate about how far it can realistically go and just what should be allowed. This issue is far too important to be decided by paternalistic scientists or governments (who appear to believe that the public are better off not knowing and not being directly involved in decision making) or even authorities initiated to regulate current activities, who appear to accept the validity of embryo research for the future. It is acknowledged that HUFEA do provide public consultation on some issues (although from previous experience it is not always well advertised), and it is unclear how much weight such responses may carry. Their Annual Reports (1994, 1995 and 1996) demonstrates the decisions taken on controversial issues and this may reflect some public opinion.

There are also issues of ownership of intellectual property to be raised including the option that such information may become protected using patents, and what access society may have to it. Would such protection of knowledge affect availability of 'treatments' in a commercial market, or would it be accessible to all? Either way, one has to consider the role and function of the embryo, in both developing and implementing these new technologies.

Many of the therapies discussed are futuristic but, with the rate of change accelerating beyond reasonable comprehension, it is impossible to predict how soon they may become available needing multi disciplinary analysis and possibly further legislation to regulate them.

Somatic cell line therapy may offer very positive opportunities for individuals and, as discussed, will hold few ethical concerns for the competent adult. However what of the fetus and embryo? What choices will prospective parents be faced with? For individual parents, who will be at the centre (if not necessarily in control) of these revolutionary techniques, reproductive choices will become broader and more complex than ever before. Speculation, which is all that can be done at present, suggests that parents planning a pregnancy will have 'life' choices to make for their future children. It must be acknowledged at this point that possibly as many as one in three pregnancies are unplanned at present (Family Planning Association, 1995, although they do admit to difficulties in accurately pinpointing this figure).

For couples at serious risk of producing children with debilitating diseases, genetic manipulation does offer a safer, if more clinical, way to achieving healthy children. However consideration must be given to just how many parents would be prepared to go through a fairly arduous journey, which is still full of potential problems – IVF treatment is still only successful in about 10–15 per cent of cases (Winston, 1994; HUFEA Annual Reports, 1994, 1995 and 1996)

Once knowledge of genes and gene sequences becomes available, how should one decide which genes to alter? Will parents be able to consider making their children taller or more intelligent? If the technology is available, would it be immoral to withhold it, based on some socially constructed criteria focused on the needs of one generation or a section of society? As for the fetus and embryo, their status may lie in the balance of just what will be allowed in the future.

CHAPTER FIVE

Infertility Treatments and Genetic Engineering

Introduction

It is important to acknowledge that, at present, any of the therapies offered by genetic engineering may involve in vitro fertilization (IVF) and selection of embryo/s for transfer to the uterus for growth and development. Such techniques, currently used in infertility treatments, have a very low success rate and this fact has to be taken into consideration when discussing the possibilities for gene therapy. The Human Fertilization and Embryology Authority (HUFEA) Annual Report (1996) demonstrated that the success rate remains low despite numerous research projects to develop the techniques. In 1985 treatments resulted in a Clinical Pregnancy Rate of 11.2 per cent and subsequent Live Birth Rate of 8.6 per cent. In 1994 the figures had only risen to 17.6 per cent for Clinical Pregnancy and 14.1 per cent for Live Birth Rate per treatment cycle (HUFEA, 1996).

In 1990, Ferguson suggested that such therapies may be possible without IVF – theoretically it may be possible to recover early fertilized human eggs, to manipulate them and re implant them in the uterus. However he does concede that in practice 'the logistics of such operations are quite mind-blowing' with current technology (Ferguson, 1990, p. 6). Therefore, even if geneticists are able to successfully achieve human gene therapy techniques, a long precarious road lies ahead for the developing embryo and fetus. This highlights the need for multidisciplinary involvement in any proposed regulations for these therapies. One also has to consider just how many parents would be willing to undergo such potentially traumatic therapies. Consequently these concerns necessitate some discussion about the issues surrounding infertility treatments themselves, if they are to play such a major role in genetic engineering techniques.

This chapter will focus on the techniques currently used to resolve infertility which involve the embryo. It is acknowledged that a number of therapies exist which do not impinge on the well-being of the embryo. However the concern here is with the effects of this technology on the moral and legal status of the embryo and fetus.

Firstly, it is the intention to provide an overview of the procedures under discussion. This includes the donation of gametes, fertilization outside the uterus and subsequent transfer of the embryo to the uterus. Discussion will focus mainly on the issues which will almost certainly affect the development of the embryo. This analysis will not include any in-depth consideration of whether infertility treatment is morally acceptable or not, as previous exploration suggests that if genetic engineering is to become a reality then such treatments will be necessary. Suffice to say, the main arguments against such treatments rests with those who, for religious or moral reasons, find it unacceptable to interfere with nature. The main concerns relate to extra uterine conception and significantly increasing the risks of death to the embryo. There is also a feeling expressed that the world is already overpopulated and technology and resources should not be used to increase this problem. However, as Joels and Wardle (1994a) state, this does not take account of the psychological and social distress caused by infertility. The argument about whether psychological pain is as deserving as physical pain often forms the basis for these debates.

Current analysis will also consider the views of conservative thinkers, who it would appear would reject the use of such techniques either because of potential violation to the life of individual embryos, or because the embryos are created outside of the natural uterus. It is believed that the procedures being considered would not respect the embryo as a person or potential person. This opinion is formed on the basis that autonomy and consent would not be respected. There is also a significant risk of death, both pre implantation and/or via later termination of the pregnancy, if the procedures were unsuccessful. Notwithstanding that, this viewpoint is worthy of consideration because it may be that subsequent generations, who believe in the sanctity of life, may find it morally acceptable to use such technology. This may be related to the fact, as demonstrated earlier with the measles vaccine, that personal and collective moral views may vary considerably depending on individual needs and expectations.

Opposing this view is the utilitarian need that using some embryo for research may enhance the well-being of future embryos. This may include improved infertility treatments, better genetic manipulation techniques and a greater understanding of the growth and development of the human being. All of this could lead to numerous advances and discoveries in science and medicine. The question for society is whether the sacrifice of some embryo is worthy of the potential benefits for many?

In the UK, these activities would appear to be acceptable by many and are licensed by HUFEA, who are the 'watch-dog' for the public. However, Sutton (1996) reports that many of our European neighbours have taken a more conservative view when legislating on this issue. For example, France, Germany and Norway have banned embryo research, while Sweden,

Norway and Germany forbid egg donation. This does rather suggest significantly different views on whether it is right to continue with such activities.

There is also the issue of the interests of the potential children, which will not form part of current discussion, but deserves mention here. As with many moral dilemmas related to reproduction, it is necessary to attempt to balance the needs and rights of prospective parents with those of their future child/ren. This is particularly apparent when discussing issues of 'who should have access to treatment', for example, post menopausal women and single women. The HUFEA has an expectation of its licensing ability that clinics who offer treatment take this consideration very seriously when dealing with individual cases.

The procedures

The most likely method for achieving gene therapy will be the manipulation of the early embryo. At present, this will involve in vitro fertilization, genetic profiles, possibly followed by genetically altering the embryo and subsequent implantation to the uterus (French Anderson, 1990; Braude, 1992). It is important to note here that these procedures may be used for women and couples who have been diagnosed as being infertile, as well as those who may be fertile but are concerned about their prospective child's genetic profile. This may be related to a family history of genetic abnormality or for other reasons such as the expectation of the 'perfect child' alluded to earlier.

The treatments will largely be similar, except that for fertile people procedures may be focused more on their own gametes rather than donated, although there may be instances when donated gametes may prove more appropriate. The possible procedures may involve:

- donation of sperm and ova;
- in vitro fertilization, with possible genetic manipulation;
- embryo transfer to the uterus.

Donation of sperm and ova

The process of IVF involves the harvesting of gametes in order to artificially create an embryo. This issue alone has several permeation's:

- prospective parents own sperm and ova
- donated sperm and own ova
- donated ova and own sperm
- donated ova and sperm.

Sperm donation is a relatively easy procedure with few risks to the man. However harvesting ovum involves firstly a technique known as Super Ovulation. This is where hormone treatment is used to stimulate the ovaries to produce several ova in the same menstrual cycle (normally only one ovum is produced). The ova are then collected either by inserting a needle, guided by ultrasound, into the vagina or by passing a laparoscope through the abdominal wall (Sutton, 1993).

In vitro fertilization

These techniques have advanced significantly in recent years and involve mixing the ovum with the sperm, which has been treated with prepared proteins, in a petri dish or test tube. With infertility treatment, the fertilized ovum is returned to the uterus once the cells have begun to divide (Steinbock, 1992; Sutton, 1993). Currently embryo selection is a fairly crude process using microscopic observation to select the most healthy looking embryo to be transferred to the uterus. The hope with genetic engineering would involve genetic profiling of the fertilized ova to determine their suitability for transfer, or for genetic manipulation before transfer. The possible processes for genetic therapy have been discussed in Chapter 1 and will not be repeated here. It is important to reiterate again that even then there is no guarantee of normality for the developing embryo/embryos, as they still have many developmental 'hurdles' to cross before birth.

Embryo transfer to the uterus

At present, there are a number of techniques used to transfer the fertilized ovum back to the mother's uterus for growth and development. Gamete Intra Fallopian Transfer (GIFT) is used in infertility treatment, although as it involves the transfer of pre fertilized sperm and ova, it may not be useful here as genetic therapy is favoured on the fertilized ovum at present.

The two commonest methods used may be Pronuclear Tubal Transfer (PROST) and Tubal Embryo Transfer (TEST). Both these procedures have been developed from GIFT and involve the transfer of an embryo, or several embryo, to the fallopian tubes. PROST occurs soon after fertilization, whereas with TEST the embryo have developed further, possibly making it a more suitable procedure following genetic manipulation (Sutton, 1993). However they both involve the need for the woman to have a general anaesthetic and laparoscopy to carry out the transfer, with some risk to both mother and embryo. Joels and Wardle (1994a) also report that their success rates are lower than GIFT techniques.

Donation of sperm and ova

When the genetic parents are the planned social parents there appears to be few ethical concerns with the process. However there are a number of ethical and legal issues to be considered when the gametes are donated. The most significant issue is related to the unique ability of sperm and ova to carry inheritance factors from one generation to another, with little control over future events. Donation of genetic material, in the form of gametes, is an individual moral decision and as such this discussion will focus on the issues following a decision to donate. The main areas for consideration are access to donors, risks to donors, identity, screening and payment.

Access to donors

According to HUFEA (1996) male donors tend to come from student populations and older men who have a family and wish to help others. Currently female donors tend to be women who have children themselves and wish to help others achieve a similar goal. They also come from women who are being sterilized or in response to publicity in the press. Donation may also come from 'spare ova' left over after successful infertility treatment (HUFEA, 1995). At the time of donation the donor can specify whether their gametes are used for research and/or infertility treatment. However they have no rights beyond this point i.e. they cannot determine who may have access to their gametes for treatment, such as a specific social class, race, sexual orientation or age group.

There is a major shortage of ova for use in infertility treatment and scientists have been exploring other avenues for ova retrieval. One of these being donated ovarian tissue from either aborted fetuses or female cadaver. This option created controversy when HUFEA (1994) produced a public consultation document to consider the viability of such procedures. In 1995, the Authority reported that following consideration of extensive responses it concluded that it was only acceptable to use live donors for infertility treatment. However they did approve the use of ovarian tissue from live, cadaver and aborted fetuses for embryo experimentation, subject to existing controls i.e. that they will be destroyed following research (HUFEA, 1995). This does create concern for the future because if these practices are considered acceptable for research, they may become acceptable for treatment in the future on a 'slippery slope' concern.

The main apprehension lies with the uniqueness of the genetic dictionary compared with other body tissue and the risk of unknown and unforeseen abnormal factors which may be inherited. Another major concern is the risk of psychological damage to the subsequent children whose genetic mother may have been a dead woman or child, or an aborted fetus. There is no way of predicting the potential damage to children who may result from this route. These concerns have largely been dismissed by writers such as Berkowitz (1995) on the basis that adopted children and children from live donors do not suffer psychologically. However at a conference in 1994 (*Who Should have Children? Who Should be Born?* London), Parsons suggested that these therapies are too new to know the full extent of the effects, psychological or otherwise, on these children. He also stated that an organization was being formed in the USA to support children who were born as a result of Artificial Insemination by Donor (AID). Surely the need for such an organization suggests some concerns about these techniques? Consequently, when the issue of cadaver and fetal tissue made headline news, there appeared to be a great deal of unease and discomfort about the idea, which may have led to such a significant response to HUFEA's (1994) consultation.

Consent to the use of ovarian tissue is another area of concern. Will women who choose to terminate a pregnancy be faced with a request to use fetal tissue for research? One has to consider how impartial or informed such consent could be at such a potentially emotional time for women. There may also be a need for women who carry Donor cards or are on the Donor Register to have an 'exclusion order' over their ovaries if they do not want them to be used for such activities.

Risks to donors

Another major issue for donors relate to the potential risks involved. As stated earlier there are few physical risks for men, but the whole issue of Super Ovulation does create concern for women. Super Ovulation can have some severe side effects. In a limited number of cases women have suffered stroke, cardiac arrest, hydatidiform moles and ovarian cancer (Sutton, 1993). If the woman has intercourse during the treatment she also increases her chances of having a multiple pregnancy, which could lead to greater health risks for both herself and the fetuses, if she decides to keep the pregnancy. One of the issues she may face is selective fetocide, if she is carrying more than two fetuses. This was sadly but clearly demonstrated in the summer of 1996 when the case of Mandy Allwell made the headlines, carrying eight fetuses, all of whom died at or shortly after birth at 19 weeks gestation (Warwick, 1996). Her anguish at originally being asked to terminate some of the fetus and later having lost them all clearly demonstrated the psychological, as well as physical risks involved. The question then has to be asked as to whether these treatments should be allowed or not? Sutton (1993) reports that some American and French centres have stopped using Super Ovulation treatment and they boast similar results as those who do.

Identity and screening

Currently donors remain anonymous. Personal information is recorded (name and date of birth) and stored at both the local clinic and at the HUFEA headquarters. They also record non identifying information such as hair colour, eye and skin colour, physical characteristics, blood group, occupation and interests. This is intended to help match donors, but no results are guaranteed. Storage of personal information does raise some concerns about future access to information. Legally, at present, recipients (and any resulting children) of donated gametes have no access to this information. This means that there is no paternity/maternity redress on the donor. Notwithstanding that, concern has to be expressed in the light of the 1975 changes to the adoption law (Jenkins, 1995) regarding access of information to birth certificates. This is particularly true if, in the future, children conceived using AID could demonstrate legitimate reasons for access to information about their genetic parents.

Concern also exists about the suitability of donor material. All donors are currently tested for sexually transmitted diseases, including Hepatitis and HIV. Screening for HIV involves freezing the sperm for six months and re-testing the donor. However genetic screening appears to be in the form of questions, rather than tests at present. HUFEA does warn potential donors that a child may be able to sue the donor if he is born with a genetic disability as a result of the donor's failure to disclose information about inherited diseases. This does put some onus on the donor to have a genetic profile performed before donation, however little information is provided in the literature on how to go about this or even if it should be done (HUFEA, 1995 and 1996). HUFEA (1995) also state that should such a case be proved then the identity of the donor could be released.

Another issue is the number of times a single donor can donate his or her gametes. The concern here would be the risk of subsequent children meeting in later life and possibly marrying a genetic brother or sister. Currently donors have to declare previous donations, and the clinics involved can check this information. However it does rely somewhat on the integrity of the donor. Assuming that children are made aware of their genetic beginnings, some may wish to prove or disprove any risk of genetic links because of the potential risks to any subsequent children from consanguinity. To minimize this risk HUFEA will provide information to individuals regarding any genetic relationship or not, but this does not involve the disclosure of personal information.

Payment

There is also the question of payment for donations to be considered. Payment was originally excluded from the 1990 HF&E Act (Section 12 (e)). This was largely intended to satisfy the notion of the donation being a gift rather than for any financial gain. There was also a risk of unscrupulous donors using the system if payment was substantial. It was equally intended to limit the risk of potential donors being subjected to pressure or excessive inducement (HUFEA, 1995). In addition to this, in July 1991, HUFEA issued a directive which allowed donors to be paid up to £15 per donation plus 'reasonable expenses'. However, with increasing demands for gametes for infertility treatment and research, it is important to keep the donation in perspective. Women need be aware of the physical risks and men and women need to be aware of the potential problems which the future may hold.

In vitro fertilization, genetic engineering and embryo transfer

The main ethical concerns about IVF relate to 'respect for the embryo'. Religious and other moral concerns focus on the notion of creating human life outside the uterus, including its attendant risks. The issues that cause most concern appear to be those affecting the embryos who are not transferred to the uterus. They may be used in research, destroyed or simply left to deteriorate in frozen limbo. Such consequences hardly respect their individual right to life or potential personhood. As these issues have been explored in Chapter 2 they will not be repeated here. Suffice to say that generally the techniques to be discussed here would largely be regarded by conservative thinkers as disrespectful, on the basis that many embryos are created which are not going to be transferred to the uterus for a chance to grow and develop (Moore, 1996).

Genetic profiling

The idea of genetic profiling is to enable parents (or the scientists involved) to choose the healthiest embryo for implantation. Moore explains the current practices in pre implantation diagnosis of genetic disorders as involving 'the removal of a single cell from a four cell embryo, or two cells from an eight cell embryo on day two; or biopsy of the trophectoderm (cells destined to become the placenta) from the five day old embryo, containing about 200 cells' (1996, p. 10). These cells could in the future have a full genetic profile carried out, and subsequent manipulation of the genes as necessary, or as is possible.

Moore (1996) reports that this procedure, currently used to test for known genetic disorders, has created some errors in diagnosis. In the USA one in five pregnancies which were supposed to carry Cystic Fibrosis free embryos were later proved to have the disorder. Stern and Alton reported in 1996 that animal studies on gene therapy for Cystic Fibrosis are progressing well. However it would appear that significant improvements in the diagnostic techniques need to be developed before they can be tested on human embryo. Consequently the gap between diagnosis and treatment needs to be narrowed further before any of these therapies became a reality (Moore, 1996). It does offer some hope for the future, especially for couples who may be at a high risk of having children with severe genetic disabilities, but consideration has to be given to just how many couples would be prepared to take up this option for other genetically linked factors.

Regarding success rates of pre implantation genetic profiling, Moore (1996) also states that one in seven fetuses were wrongly diagnosed female and were later aborted because of this!

Sex selection

The whole issue of sex selection deserves a mention here, as this is one of the many issues which genetic profiling may create. There appears to be two main reasons for parents wishing to know the sex of their embryo or fetus. One is related to the risk of X linked genetic disorders, which can be severe and debilitating (depending on the extent of the effects). The other is choice. The concern with choice usually rests with the assumption that most parents (with some exceptions) may choose male over female, creating an imbalance in society. Hoskins and Holmes (1984) argued that some may see sex selection as a more sophisticated form of family planning. For women and couples, in particular circumstances, it may be appropriate – the family already has three females and desperately long for a male or visa versa, the woman who would care for only female or only male children. It has to be said that the legitimacy of these requests may be questioned, and would deserve careful consideration and analysis before proceeding.

So the question goes 'should "ordinary" people be allowed such choices?'. Hoskins and Holmes (1984) go on to counter argue this point on the basis that history and research clearly demonstrate that the majority would choose a male first-born. This is related to long held social beliefs and perceptions of the positive benefits of having a first born male. This belief was reiterated by Mosher (1993), writing about China's one child policy, where they now have a major shortage of females. Sangari (1984), writing about the social, religious and economic importance of sons in India, further demonstrates the point.

The embryo/fetus as a commodity?

Once the embryo/s have been transferred back to the uterus, they still remain at risk from interference. If parents are focused on having a 'normal' child they may well choose to have prenatal diagnostic tests to assess the progress and success of development. If they demonstrate the fetus is suffering from a disorder or potential disorder they may well then choose to terminate the pregnancy and try again. This, to a certain extent, demonstrates the ability of the embryo and fetus to become a commodity, which if defective can be destroyed. It also says little about their humanness or potential to be a person. The issue of termination may be further complicated if the woman is carrying more than one live fetus. There are two scenarios to be considered. Firstly, if one fetus is 'normal' he may be put at risk if parents choose to destroy the 'abnormal' one. Secondly, if the parents were planning for one child, they may be faced with the decision to terminate one or more of the surviving embryos. The risks to mother and fetuses of a multiple pregnancy are clearly documented, however parents may find the dilemma of which fetus to terminate an unexpected complication. There is always a risk of losing all, or terminating some healthy fetuses, only to later discover that the 'one that was saved' is not perfect. The psychological effects of such decision making are enormous, and parents would need to be fully aware of all the consequences before embarking on such a journey (Joels and Wardle, 1994b).

Mason (1990) suggests that the notion of taking some lives in order to improve/save others is generally repugnant, but it may be difficult to justify the 'severe mental trauma and the economic waste involved in preserving large numbers of fetuses in the near certainty that they will die as neonates' (Mason, 1990, p. 71). He is, of course, referring to high multiple pregnancy. However in 1996 the media reported great concern when an obstetrician admitted to selective fetocide practices on healthy twins to preserve the mother's psychological well-being (Cooper, *The Independent*, 5th August). Consideration has to be given to the extent of the outcry which followed, especially as, according to the latest figures, some 172,069 fetuses were terminated in 1992 (OPCS, 1995), a significant number of which would have been for similar reasons. Perhaps society is uneasy with the notion of choice in these cases. How does one reconcile making the right choice over two or more apparently healthy fetuses?

As demonstrated, IVF and embryo transfer will inevitably increase the risks of death to the pre implanted embryo. It may also increase the number of therapeutic abortion and so will do little to protect the 'rights' of the embryo and fetus. Again the question is asked, who is entitled to have their rights recognized the most? The embryo, the fetus, the woman/parents or indeed the scientists?

The conservative viewpoint

The aforementioned techniques involve the manipulation of gametes external to the uterus with the intention of creating a new person or potential person. Liberal thinkers would argue that these cells amount to neither yet, but to something that may develop into a person at sometime in the future. Therefore it would appear that the use of these therapies assumes some, if not total, acceptance that the pre implantation embryo has no intrinsic value. 'It' is only valuable for 'its' ability to be useful as a subject for research to improve the outcome of subsequent embryos and human beings.

The difference between teachings and practice

The Catholic Church, seen to hold conservative views, disagree with some infertility treatments, not just because of the rights of the unborn, but they argue against assisted conception on the basis that procreation should not be separated from sexual intercourse (Kearon, 1995). This argument is also used to defend their position on contraception. However what is taught and practised are not always congruent. This was illustrated in a recent report from the USA on abortion figures, by the Alan Guttmacher Institute (Rovner, 1996). It demonstrated that the main reason for American women seeking abortion was failure of contraception (57.5 per cent), and that one in five stated their religious beliefs as Evangelical or Born Again Christian, while 31.3 per cent were Roman Catholic – all of whom would appear to disagree with abortion if following the teachings of their particular chosen religion.

The discarded embryos

The main problem for conservative thinkers generally appears to be the discarded embryo, the ones which are created and not implanted. At present these embryos are created in vitro and many philosophers would argue that it is better to exist than not (Glover et al., 1989), especially as transfer to the uterus does provide an opportunity for growth and development. The options for those who are not chosen include:

1. They may be frozen for later use, either if treatment is unsuccessful, or the couple choose to have more children. However freezing can damage them and some, if not all, may perish.
2. They may be used in research, as a means to an end for others, but have no real value in themselves.
3. They may be destroyed and some would argue that it is a total waste of their creation, if they are not used at all (Glover et al., 1989).
4. They may be donated to another woman who is having infertility treatment.

Either of the first three options increases the risks of destruction of the embryo, whilst the fourth carries its own moral dilemmas, similar to those discussed earlier about donation. In conclusion the conservative thinker has little option but to reject these therapies if the moral rights of the embryo and fetus are to be considered seriously, on the basis of his ability to become a thinking moral person.

Conclusion

Technology will proceed at a rate of success that is difficult to predict. The use of these therapies would appear to have little real concern for the well-being of the embryo as an individual potential person. The potential value for the human race is vast, especially if HUGO's promise to attempt to lessen the many stresses caused by debilitating genetic disorders and genetically linked diseases comes true, and this should not be denied. However, it must be tempered with the caution of 'how far is it prepared to go?' or 'how far will individual societies allow it to go?'.

At present, the embryo is legally protected after the 14 day limit from research, yet it is the first four days that genetic engineers are concerned with. The number of embryo who may perish in this process of discovery is unknown, but could be enormous. An unknown holocaust all of its own! Consideration also has to be given for the need for more donated gametes as science moves forward. Will society be prepared to continue, and increase, their gamete donations for research and genetic engineering purposes? It must be remembered that current donation has the emphasis on 'the gift of a child'.

The whole issue of cadaver and aborted fetal tissue will be debated again, as the need for more ova increases. Perhaps it will become more acceptable with its use in research. After all IVF in 1978–79 caused many moral dilemmas at the time, the idea of conception in a tube was not accepted positively by all. Yet now, it is 'simply' part of infertility treatment, which is extensively used and does not make headline news in the way it did then.

The prospective parents will need extensive counselling before proceeding with any of the proposals, especially as their expectations of success may be much greater than the reality. The current 14.1 per cent live birth rate (HUFEA, 1996) may not be encouraging and it does not include the number of discarded embryo or unsuccessful attempts from current therapies. For parents, the reality of disappointment and the financial and emotional stress may be greater than anticipated, and has to be catered for in any developments.

It is reasonable to speculate that such potentially traumatic therapies may well be considered worse for some couples than accepting infertility or current alternatives to gene therapy. However for many couples this may offer a reasonable and acceptable chance of having 'normal' children and as the therapies are being developed, it could be considered morally unacceptable by many not to proceed and hope for better success. Notwithstanding that, the recurrent and haunting concern remains as to how far society or science could go or would be willing to go.

CHAPTER SIX

Genetics, the Fetus and the Future

Introduction

The complexities of intimately knowing our genetic makeup and consequently something of our future has not yet begun to unravel. It is predicted to affect parts of our lives that we cannot begin to comprehend at present. The genome exists – it can be seen and split, and already this knowledge is being applied to diagnosis, possible treatments and preventative measures for disease states caused by genes and gene sequences. It is also acknowledged that genes are not the only determining factor in development of disease and that environment and other factors may affect one's predisposition towards some illness. How long before it will be possible to distinguish hair or eye colour, stature or level of potential intelligence? How long before embryonic profiles can predict the risks and realities of diseases that may develop in later life? And what will medicine be able to do with these predictions?

The answers to these questions lie in the future and exciting though it all sounds, it has to be tempered with cautionary analysis of the effects this may have on the future of the human race. This applies particularly to the legal and moral fate of the fetus and embryo. The focus in this concluding chapter will be towards the future, in particular, relating to whether this knowledge explosion will affect our thinking about the development of personhood and the impact of any such changes on legislation relating to the fetus and embryo. This will involve a focus on the slippery slope arguments and how realistic they are. It will also continue with issues relating to the legal status of the embryo and fetus in the future.

Embryo research is practised at present and the developments from the human genome initiative appear to ensure a need for such activities in the future. Therefore it would appear that protecting these embryos from this utilitarian work may no longer be within our capacity. There can be no going back in science and technology – progress can be justified and the future may hold discoveries that will enhance and improve man(woman) kind. However that does not give open licence to continue without appropriate regulation and control by multidisciplinary teams (and international cooperation). Such regulation should include the limits of research and protection against discrimination, in particular eugenic practices which may appear to benefit some sections of society. Attempts should also be made to maintain openness and accurate education about the realities of what can and cannot be achieved, if confusion and scaremongering are to be minimized. Is it inevitable that such a significant knowledge explosion will affect our current values and beliefs about the moral and legal status of the fetus and embryo?

The human genome and the slippery slope

The Human Genome knowledge will add to our understanding of how we function and behave. In itself it is a relatively harmless, if expensive exercise in developing human knowledge. Having said this, the discovery by Hamer in 1993 of a gene that may be linked to homosexuality sparked some controversy with headlines such as 'Homosexual gene test not far off' (Redford, *The Guardian*, 23rd February, 1994). However the projects are advancing with specific purposes in mind and it is this agenda which appears to be causing excitement and concern. The idea that society could control or eliminate some of the devastating diseases currently inherited is very alluring. Notwithstanding that, there is concern about how illness/disability is defined, which in turn leads to concerns about how far this new knowledge could be used to alter individuals or subsequent generations of individuals, in terms of eugenic practices.

Ledley (1994) provides a useful discussion in an attempt to distinguish genetics from eugenics. He uses Rawl's theory of 'justice as fairness' to defend the idea that *genetics* is concerned with improving the lot of individuals, which is acceptable and just, whilst *eugenics* is concerned with societies. He argues that any new technology should be applied to 'extending individual liberties and be applied to the greatest benefit of individuals with the least advantages' (Ledley, 1994, p. 157), those who suffer or have the potential to suffer severe disabilities. Eugenics, being concerned with societies, may be used to reinforce prejudice and discrimination by using *positive eugenics* (to enhance those already considered to be superior in intelligence, race, behaviour etc.) or *negative eugenics* (involving discrimination against the reproduction of those with perceived disabilities). Interestingly Resnick (1994) defines negative eugenics as that of eliminating disease rather than discrimination – it would seem that the same term may be used in conjunction with individuals or societies. The assumption made about eugenics appears to be that only 'perfect people' will survive, but as already discussed, no one has come up with a definition of the 'perfect person' yet!

A major concern raised by these practices is that society may be embarking on the biggest slippery slope ever, in an attempt to create a 'Brave New (more perfect) World'. Such 'slippery slope' arguments exist consistently in ethics, the idea that if society allows A to happen for a legitimate and positive cause, then B will follow as acceptance of A becomes the norm within society. This has been demonstrated with prenatal screening tests to diagnose fetal abnormalities – as tests become more sophisticated and safer, parents have higher expectations of having 'normal' children and the uptake of such tests have increased over recent years. This may, in part, be due to the fact that families are much smaller now, therefore there is a greater need to 'get it right' first time and social pressures may also reinforce this need. Many authors (Richards and Green, 1993) now suggest that for the majority of women screening the fetus has become part of normal antenatal care. This has led to a reduction in the number of children born with conditions such as neural tube defect and Down's Syndrome, through the process of screening, diagnosis and termination of the pregnancy (Green and Richards, 1993). Is this not a subtle form of eugenics by elimination?

The 'advantage' genetic engineering would possibly have over current technology would be to eliminate the need for later pregnancy termination and as such may be viewed as acceptable by some. This would not necessarily improve the status of the embryo but may enhance the status of the fetus by lowering the risks of termination for fetal abnormality. It is possible that the fetus would then gain status through arguments suggesting that aborting the fetus up to 24 weeks is no longer acceptable, as parents have the advantage of early diagnosis and possible manipulation and/or selective implantation of the embryo. However it has to be remembered that in 1992 (the most recent statistics available) there were 172,069 abortions carried out in England and Wales, only 1,828 of those being associated with a medical condition in the fetus (OPCS, 1995). Therefore the effects may be limited. However, in time, it may be possible for pro-life activists to argue successfully for a general lowering of the 24 week limit using this increased status as an argument against destroying such advanced fetuses.

Regardless of this speculation, consideration has to be given to this apparent social need for 'normal' healthy children in terms of a real or imagined slippery slope for future genetics (Krimsky and Hubbard, 1995). Previous discussion focused on the socially constructed need for normality, and it also appears to take the form of attempting to restrict the practices of pregnant women. Field (1989) reported, from the USA, on moves to control the behaviour of women who smoke or abuse alcohol and other drugs. She suggested that it is not beyond reason to justify forcing women to have prenatal diagnostic tests that may influence pregnancy termination decisions or even legally force them to have fetal surgery to protect and enhance their fetuses chances for normality.

The issue here is concerned with how far society may be prepared to go to produce the 'normal healthy' child eluded to. However, this again brings up the issue of defining normal! How many fetuses may be put at risk by mothers frightened of the authorities and reluctant to seek help if they fear coercion, and how many fetuses may be terminated because they do not meet this socially constructed criteria for normality? There is an anxiety that two slippery slopes run side by side – the fetus as a human entity with moral values will probably inevitably be affected by progress in genetic engineering, as the fetus loses moral significance, genetic engineering may increase or visa versa!

Rifkin (cited in Holtug, 1993) sums up the slippery slope proponents of human gene therapy thus:

> 'Once we decide to begin the process of human genetic engineering, there is really no logical place to stop. If diabetes, sickle cell anaemia, and cancer are cured by altering the genetic makeup of an individual, why not proceed to other "disorders": myopia, colour-blindness, left-handedness? Indeed, what is to preclude a society from deciding that a certain skin colour is a disorder?'

However, Holtug (1993) argues that provided society maintains the boundary between *'corrective genetic therapy'* and *'enhancement'* therapy, the slippery slope argument fails but this could only be achieved through regulation and control. Resnick (1994) also argues against slippery slope concerns when he looks specifically at germ line gene therapy (as opposed to somatic cell therapy) and suggests that genetic enhancement need not be unethical or unjust, if properly regulated and accompanied by adequate education. His line of thinking is assuming that education will dispel fears and lessen prejudice and discrimination. However the value of education in creating social change can be challenged based on past and present experiences. The traditional view of Health Education can be represented thus:

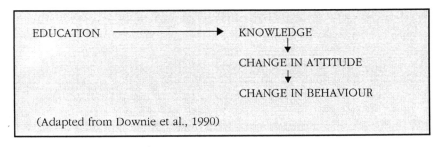

(Adapted from Downie et al., 1990)

Fig. 6.1

It involves the notion that education will increase knowledge and understanding, which will create a change in attitude leading to behavioural transformations. However health promotion experts (Downie et al., 1990; Beattie et al., 1993; Webb, 1994) are now looking at different models for changing behaviour because education alone is not working. An example of this failure is the recent Health of the Nation report which suggest that smoking, especially among women and teenagers, continues to rise despite the widespread campaigns about the potential hazards (Calman, 1994).

Another issue to be considered is the risk of creating further discrimination towards people who have had genetic engineering therapy as opposed to those who have not. While Resnick argues that such therapies need not take from genetically engineered individuals' dignity or self worth, he does concede that it 'may cause harm to unengineered people by contributing to existing prejudices and social stigma' (1994, p. 37). He also remains concerned that the main reason for germ line therapy should be prevention of genetic disease with a secondary reason of genetic enhancement.

The overriding issue in managing these slippery slope concerns appears to be the need for control, including a focus on who should have that control – governments, scientists or specialist agencies? Who could be viewed as having the best interests of society and future generations uppermost in its deliberations? The objective option may be for a specialist multidisciplinary agency, with the power and democracy to represent pluralistic views.

How real is the issue of a slippery slope for the embryo? The status of the pre embryo suggests an attempt to consider the early embryo as cells to be used as raw material in experimentation to produce a more perfect being, and it would appear that supporters of such research already believe this. Speculation then has to question whether such research would stop at the 14 day limit! One of the reasons for this limit is because the primitive streak develops soon after, when it may be possible for the embryo to feel pain. Supposing research led to safe anaesthesia or analgesia for the embryo, what would stop later experimentation being accepted and legislated for? What of the status of the embryo then? Would the embryo become known as a pre fetus, suggesting something less than developing human being?

Another question to be considered is whether this society can possibly know how future generations may react to such therapies? The answer to this may only lie in the future, as previous generations failed to predict current day reactions to controversial issues such as slavery, human and animal torture and abuse of the environment. Admittedly this was through ignorance of the knowledge that has been developed today, however will the present society be viewed as equally primitive by future generations? We cannot begin to predict how such decisions may be viewed in 2050 or beyond.

Previous discussion has also demonstrated the difficulties of consensus opinion when living in a pluralist society, where some sections consider experimentation of embryos as being in the best interests of others, despite any concerns about slippery slopes, whilst other members of the same society object categorically to any interference with the growing embryo and fetus. However, lack of consensus may not prevent a shift in the collective morality of a society. It could be argued that it is already happening as acceptance of the right to abortion and other comparable issues proliferate (e.g. euthanasia), while pro life organizations and similar groups are seen as minority groups in today's society.

Women's rights are often cited in this debate and one has to consider whether they have to be seen in opposition to the fetus. The right to free, available, safe abortion is considered to form a significant part of the process of improving women's status worldwide. However consideration has to be given to the rights of the fetus and embryo, preferably without detracting from the validity of rights for women for respect as equal members of society, for good safe lifestyles, equal access to education, health care and employment etc. Do reproductive rights (i.e. access to contraception, infertility treatments etc.) always have to include the right to destroy the fetus?

As demonstrated, some authors try to debunk the slippery slope argument (Holtug, 1993; Resnick., 1994; Agar, 1995), but it always appears to return to the same issue of how far individuals or specific societies are prepared to go!

The legal status of the embryo and the fetus in the future

The legal status of the fetus and embryo demonstrates that quite diverse laws co-exist within society. The developments in genetic engineering will create other opportunities for legal constraints, but will they affect the mother, fetus or professional more? It would appear that there will be a need for collective responsibility between mothers and professionals (Knoppers, 1993), but there is still the issue of who will have the control – the mother or the professional? It is possible to speculate that the professional involved may have most control, with the fate of an individual fetus within the control of the mother, but what of the fate of other fetuses, embryos and gametes?

Based on earlier discussion it would appear that as gametes are not considered potential persons then the genome would be treated in a similar way by legislation. The genome, it seems, will be treated as a cell and as such pre human and not worthy of a legal protection or only limited regulation. For this reason, it may be possible to conduct experiments on the genome without further legislation. However, there is an issue of the experimented on gamete being fertilized and implanted for growth. The

HF&E Act (1990) states that 'a licence... cannot authorize altering the genetic structure of any cell while it forms part of an embryo' but what is to stop manipulation before fertilization and then subsequent implantation of that embryo? Currently the HF&E Act (1990) does not allow experimented-on embryos to be implanted, as they have to be discarded before the primitive streak appears. However, if the 'procedure' was considered as a 'therapy' (therapy could be defined for the benefit of that embryo, whereas experimentation would be concerned with research generally) and not experimentation, then it may be possible to proceed without further legislation. Schedule 2 of the Act (HF&E Act, 1990) specifies that embryos must be in a suitable condition to be implanted, therefore under current legislation it would be necessary to demonstrate their suitability for implantation before proceeding.

Any further legal changes will depend on just what may be possible or permissible. Speculation leads to consideration of the extreme options.

1. **Experimentation on the embryo will be considered unnecessary and become outlawed, in which case the HF&E Act (1990), in its current form, would have to be abolished with different legislation being introduced to replace it.**
   Sadly, from a fetal and embryonic perspective, this seems highly unlikely at present, as the advances made can be justified, even though many are not necessarily involved with life threatening diseases (e.g. infertility treatments, contraception and miscarriage). It is acknowledged that these problems can cause significant psychological trauma, but generally do not threaten life, and perhaps the focus should be on alternative methods of treatment. It may appear to be a radical move considering the reported success in using embryo research, but if the fetus and embryo are to survive into the next century with some dignity and respect this may be the only reasonable option!

2. **Genetic engineering on human beings will continue, which could lead to abuses of genetic manipulation practices in attempts to produce 'perfect' people, according to social or parental specification. If legislation is not there to protect the vulnerable fetus and embryo, then what is to stop excessive experimentation, manipulation and destruction of embryos who do not meet agreed acceptable specifications? The term acceptable could refer to a variety of desired traits – again the issue of who will decide on these?**
   There are legal obligations to protect children, the Children Act (1989) has to a certain extent protected them against today's society, not just because they are vulnerable but because they are an investment in the future. Is it then reasonable to want to protect the children who are not yet born?

The answer to this probably depends on whether these new technologies are considered sufficiently beneficial to be allowed. Attention will also need to be directed towards the rights of the fetus and/or those of the mother. The whole issue of maternal autonomy has been eluded to and will almost certainly be linked to professional control of just which therapies will be offered (Schwartz Cowan, 1993). This is an area of considerable interest and the objective system would provide for professional and mother in an equal partnership. However if the professional holds the finance and the technology, what of the mothers' autonomy for decision making etc?

Dixon (1993) states that we may be among the last generations to have uninterrupted inheritance. However one has to consider just how many people would actually use such therapies and this should form a significant part of any debate relating to continuing with embryo research. Will it be an elitist minority who may use them, in which case should such significant resources be used on embryo experimentation to develop the technology?

The concern is that, as in the past, with laws on abortion, the legally unprotected fetus and embryo may be predisposed to the social concerns of the day rather than being accepted for who he may become. One example of the reality of this can be seen in China today, with their one child per family policy. Mosher (1993) provides a graphic description of the problems which exist with a strict regime of family planning control, where not only termination of pregnancy is encouraged but infanticide and wilful neglect of female babies is also reported. Research is now showing a gross shortage of girls and women because if populations are limited in such a manner people choose to have sons. What if people can choose hair colour, skin colour, temperament, freedom from disease states – what future for the fetus and embryo if not protected by some form of legal framework? In making such decisions, greater problems may develop than can be predicted at present. It may take a long time to know all the capacities and limitations of genes and gene sequences. Therefore attention needs to be focused now on the acceptable practices and those which should be outlawed in legislation. Future legislation would also have to provide a flexible element to allow for unforeseen consequences with a review of developments and advances (at least annually), which is currently part of the remit of HUFEA. As for the embryo and fetus, it would appear to depend on whether the majority or most vociferous group of the day believe in his right to legal protection from use and abuse.

Will the human genome knowledge explosion affect our individual and collective beliefs about the moral and legal status of the fetus and embryo?

Many of the therapies are futuristic. However now is the time to consider the possible consequences of continuing this research. It would appear to be too late to stop the 'roller-coaster' of knowledge and technology and it may be inappropriate to do so. The potential benefits of knowing what makes us human, what defines our possibilities and limitations could enhance personal and professional potential, enabling us to get the most out of life. This could be achieved through enabling strategies and appropriate education, as well as using the technology known as genetic engineering.

However, if our 'worst fears' are not to be realized, then there is an absolute need for regulation and appropriate control of these practices, in particular in relation to the role the fetus and embryo may play in these developments. It may be necessary to reconsider the whole issue of embryo experimentation if the embryo is to be protected from mass destruction in the name of science. However those involved and agreeable to such research may argue on the grounds that foregoing research would only drive it 'underground', with no control, and that could be even more devastating than present practices.

Another argument could be related to the numerous potential benefits attributed to the research. Watt (1993) argues that worthwhile human activities such as medicine are not just about what people want, therefore perhaps the question that needs serious consideration is 'whether these perceived benefits are about what people think they want or what they really need?'. Is perfection in all really necessary and appropriate, or can we learn to live in peace with our differences?

Despite efforts to debunk the slippery slope concerns, there is a definite sense that science and society have already embarked on a road, that has only one direction – regulation is essential if some form of protection is to be provided.

The issues of public debate, education and health promotion tactics have been raised and need further development. There is a definite need for vigilance in producing accurate factual information so that all interested parties can put forward their considered opinions – if people see the pre embryo as a human entity, would there be an outcry at the mass destruction being carried out at present, or would justification of its use win the day? All this is only possible if public debate is encouraged.

It would appear unethical to withhold information and technology that could advance medicine, but will it have to be at the expense of the embryo or pre embryo? Is it possible to shift more effort and resources to other avenues, which may take longer to develop, but would be more acceptable long term? Analysis of the evidence would appear to suggest that the Human Genome knowledge explosion will affect current moral beliefs about the human embryo, however it will not create a singular status. Those who believe that the embryo, from conception, has the potential to become a thinking moral person will continue to campaign for an end to practices which treat the embryo as less than human. These conservative thinkers may reject such therapies, as degrading and unfair to the developing human being. However, looking at the experience of the recent vaccination campaign, there may be concern that some who would consider themselves to be conservative thinkers may choose to justify the short term 'sacrifice' of some embryos for the benefit of many, in the long term!

On the other side of the divide, there are those who will continue to justify embryo experimentation, and argue that the embryo deserves no such respect, believing that such status should be reserved for the fetus or baby. It will be interesting to see how such divided attitudes could be represented in legislation, if this is possible (because it did not happen with the HF&E Act, 1990).

The issue of enhancement and eugenic practices create even more dilemmas for society. This is not just because of concerns about unknown or unprecedented side effects, but also because of the concern of creating even more discrimination in a world that has not yet learned to reconcile itself to different races, cultures and different morality.

Notwithstanding that, it could be possible for society to view the embryo as raw material to becoming a vehicle for genetic enhancement. Could he become deserving of special status because of his potential to improve his capacity for living and minimize the limitations of the 20th century human being through this genetic therapy revolution? Unfortunately this would do little to save him from experimentation and research.

It is the author's considered belief that there can be no going back in science. However now is the time to consider whether continuing with embryo research is an absolute and acceptable road to take. Attention has to be given to possible alternatives if the embryo is to maintain his current meagre status and possibly enhance his status in the future. There is a danger that if an enhanced status is not sought then he and many like him are on a slippery slope of decline to oblivion, in terms of moral significance. The danger in this is that moral status does affect legislation and other aspects of life.

It is not possible to accurately predict the positive or negative discoveries ahead, therefore appropriate multidisciplinary international alliance and consensus should be sought to control and regulate these practices. This is necessary to ensure that counter productive and adverse affects may be minimized and experimentation should be reserved for those who are in a position to consent to research. It must be remembered that whether dealing with genes, gametes or embryos, science is experimenting with one of the most precious of all entities – the human being.

References

Chapter One

Annas, G.J., Elias, S. (1993). 'Legal and ethical issues in genetic screening, prenatal diagnosis and gene therapy'. In: Simpson, J.C., Elias, S. (Eds). *Essentials of Prenatal Diagnosis*. Edinburgh: Churchill Livingstone.

Begley, S. et al. (1993). 'Cures from the womb'. *Newsweek*, 22nd February, pp. 49–51.

Blackburn, S.T., Loper, D.L. (1992). *Maternal, Fetal And Neonatal Physiology: A Clinical Perspective*. USA: WB Saunders Co.

Braude, P.R. (1992). 'Embryo therapy: what can be done?'. In: Bronham, D. et al. (Eds). *Ethics in Reproductive Medicine*. London: Springler-Verlag.

Caskey, C.T. (1993). 'DNA based medicine: prevention and therapy'. In: Kevles, D.J., Hood, L. (Eds). *The Code of Codes*. USA: Harvard University Press.

Dawson, K. (1993). 'An outline of scientific aspects of embryo research'. In: Singer, P. et al. (Eds). *Embryo Experimentation: Ethical, Legal and Social Issues*. Cambridge: Cambridge University Press.

Dixon, P. (1993). *The Genetic Revolution*. Eastbourne: Kingsway Publishers.

Elliott, R. (1993). 'Identity and the ethics of gene therapy'. *Bioethics,* Vol. 7, No. 1, pp. 27–40.

Emery, A.E.H., Mueller, R.F. (1992). *Elements of Medical Genetics*. London: Churchill Livingstone.

Ferguson, M.W.J. (1990). 'Contemporary and future possibilities for human embryonic manipulation'. In: Dyson, A., Harris, J. (Eds). *Experiments on Embryo*. London: Routledge Press.

Fletcher, S. (1992). 'Innovative treatment or ethical headache? Fetal transplantation in Parkinson's Disease'. *Professional Nurse,* June, pp. 592–595.

French Anderson, W. (1990). 'Human gene therapy: scientific and ethical considerations'. In: Chadwick, R.F. (Ed). *Ethics, Reproduction and Genetic Control*. London: Routledge Press.

Glover, J. et al. (1989). *Fertility and the Family: The Glover Report on Reproductive Technologies to the European Commission*. London: Fourth Estate Ltd.

Greely, H.T. (1993) 'Health insurance, employment discrimination and the genetic revolution'. In: Kevles, D.J., Hood, L. (Eds). *The Code of Codes*. USA: Harvard University Press.

Hawkes, N. (1994). 'The greatest discovery of our time? Genes'. *The Times,* 2 May.

Higginson, R. (1987). 'The ethics of experimentation'. In: De S. Cameron, N.M. (Ed). *Embryo's and Ethics: The Warnock Reporting Debate*. Edinburgh: Rutherford House Books.

Judson, H.F. (1993). 'A history of the science and technology behind gene mapping and sequencing'. In: Kevles, D.J., Hood, L. (Eds). *The Code of Codes*. USA: Harvard University Press.

Kevles, D.J., Hood, L. (1993). *The Code of Codes*. USA: Harvard University Press.

Morgan, D., Lee, R.G. (1991). *Blackstone's Guide to the Human Fertilization and Embryology Act 1990*. London: Blackstone Press Ltd.

Nicholl, D.S.T. (1994). *An Introduction to Genetic Engineering*. Cambridge: Cambridge University Press.

Persson, I. (1995). 'Genetic therapy, identity and the person regarding reasons'. *Bioethics,* pp. 14–31.

Rennie, J. (1994). 'Grading the gene tests'. *Scientific American,* June, pp. 64–74.

Schenker, J.G. (1992). 'The rights of the pre embryo and fetus to in-vitro and in-vivo therapy'. In: Bromham, D. et al. (Ed). *Ethics in Reproductive Medicine*. London: Springer–Verlag.

Stanworth, M. (1987). 'The deconstruction of motherhood'. *Reproductive Technologies: Gender, Motherhood and Medicine*. Cambridge: Polity Press.

Tortora, G.J., Grabowski, S.R (1993). *Principles of Anatomy and Physiology*. 7th Edition. USA: Harper Collins College Publishers.

Van De Graaff, K.M., Fox, S.I. (1989). *Concepts of Human Anatomy and Physiology*. 2nd Edition. USA: Wm. C. Brown Publishers.

Watt, H. (1993). 'Genetic intervention and the good of human beings'. *Catholic Medical Quarterly,* Vol. XLIV, No. 259, pp. 17–21.

Weatherall, D.J. (1991). *The New Genetics and Clinical Practice*. 3rd Edition. Oxford: Oxford University Press.

Chapter Two

Baird, R.M., Rosenbaum, S.E. (1989). *The Ethics Of Abortion*. New York, USA: Prometheus Books.

Finnis, J. (1973). 'The rights and wrongs of abortion: A reply to Judith Thompson'. *Contemporary Moral Problems,* pp. 68–72.

Fulford, K.W.M. et al. (1994). *Medicine and Moral Reasoning*. Cambridge: Cambridge University Press.

Gillon, R. (1985). 'To what do we have moral obligation and why?'. *British Medical Journal,* Vol. 290, 8th June, pp. 1734–1736.

Gillon, R. (1991). 'Human embryos and the argument from potential'. *Journal of Medical Ethics,* Vol. 17, pp. 59–61.

Glover, J. et al. (1989). *Fertility and the Family: The Glover Report on Reproductive Technologies to European Commission*. London: Fourth Estate Ltd.

Glover, J. (1990). *Causing Death and Saving Lives*. London: Penguin Books Ltd.

Harris, J. (1992). *The Value of Life*. London: Routledge and Kegan Paul plc.

Harris, J. (1993). *Wonderwoman and Superman: The Ethics of Human Biotechnology*. Oxford: Oxford University Press.

Hawkes, N. (1994). 'The greatest discovery of all times?'. *The Times Newspaper*, 2 May, p. 7.

Holland, A. (1990). 'A fortnight of my life is missing: a discussion of the status of the human pre embryo'. *Journal of Applied Philosophy*, Vol. 7, No. 1, pp. 25–37.

Jones, D.G. (1989). 'Brain birth and personal identity'. *Journal of Medical Ethics*, Vol. 15, pp. 173–178.

Jones, D.G., Telfer, B. (1995). 'Before I was an embryo, I was a pre embryo: or was I?'. *Bioethics*, Vol. 9, No. 1, pp. 32–49

Kohn, M. (1994). 'Stretched genes'. *The Observer Newspaper*, 6 March, p. 4.

Mappes, T.A., Zembaty, J.S. (1991). *Biomedical Ethics*. 3rd Edition. New York, USA: McGraw Hill Inc.

Moore, K.L. (1983). *Before We Are Born*. 2nd Edition. London: WB Saunders

Morgan, D., Lee, R.G. (1991). *Blackstone's Guide to the Human Fertilisation and Embryology Act 1990*. London: Blackstone Press Ltd.

Murphy, S. (1992) *Talking about Miscarriage*. London: Sheldon Press.

Neilson, J., Grant, A. (1991). 'Ultrasound in pregnancy'. In: Chalmers, I. et al. (Eds). *Effective Care in Pregnancy and Childbirth Vol. 1*. Oxford: Oxford University Press.

Noonan, H. (1991). *Personal Identity*. London: Routledge Press.

Noonan, J.T. (1991). 'An almost absolute value in history: abortion & maternal/fetal conflict'. In: Mappes, T.A., Zembaty, J.S. (Eds). *Biomedical Ethics*. 3rd Edition. New York, USA: McGraw Hill Inc.

Oakley, A. et al. (1990). *Miscarriage*. London: Penguin Books.

Pojman, L.P. (1992). *Life and Death – Grappling with the Moral Dilemmas of Our Times*. London: Jones & Bartlett Publishers.

Pojman, L.P. (1993). *Life and Death: A Reader in Moral Problems*. London: Jones & Bartlett Publishers.

Poplawski, N., Gillett, G. (1991). 'Ethics and embryos'. *Journal of Medical Ethics*, Vol. 17, pp. 62–69.

Rumbold, G. (1993). *Ethics In Nursing Practice*. 2nd Edition. London: Bailliere Tindall.

Singer, P. (1979). *Practical Ethics*. Cambridge: Cambridge University Press.

Steinbock, B. (1992). *Life Before Birth: The Moral and Legal Status of Embryos and Fetuses*. Oxford: Oxford University Press.

Thompson, J.J. (1971). 'A defence of abortion'. *Philosophy and Public Affairs*, Vol. 1, No. 1, Autumn, pp. 47–68.

Tooley, M. (1972). 'Abortion and infanticide'. *Philosophy and Public Affairs*, Vol. 2, No. 1, Autumn, pp. 37–65.

Urmson, J.O. (1994). 'Morality: invention of discovery?'. In: Fulford, K.W.M. et al. (Eds). *Medicine and Moral Reasoning*. Cambridge: Cambridge University Press.

Warnock, M. (1985). *A Question of Life*. Oxford: Basil Blackwell Ltd.

Warnock, M. (1987). 'Do human cells have rights?'. *Bioethics,* Vol. 1, No. 1, pp. 1–14.

Warren, M. A. (1991). 'On the moral and legal status of abortion'. In: Mappes, T.A., Zembaty, J.S. (Eds). *Biomedical Ethics*. 3rd Edition. New York, USA: McGraw Hill Inc.

White, V. (1994). 'The moral status of the fetus'. *Midwives Chronicle and Nursing Notes,* October, pp. 375–378.

Chapter Three

Brazier, M. (1992). *Medicine. Patients and the Law*. London: Penguin Books.

Capon, A.M. (1992). 'Parenthood and frozen embryos: more than property and privacy'. *The Hastings Centre Report*, September/October, pp. 32–33.

Dawson, K. (1993). 'An outline of scientific aspects of embryo research'. In: Singer, P. et al. (Eds). *Embryo Experimentation: Ethical, Legal and Social Issues*. Cambridge: Cambridge University Press.

Downie, R.S., Calman, K.C. (1994). *Healthy Respect*. 2nd Edition. Oxford: Oxford University Press.

Field, M.A. (1989). 'Controlling the woman to protect the fetus'. *Law, Medicine and Health Care,* Vol. 17, No. 2, Summer, pp. 114–129.

Gallagher, J. (1986). 'The fetus and the law: whose life is it anyway?'. *Childbirth Trends MIDIRS Information Pack,* Vol. 3, December.

Gaze, B. (1990). 'Public policy and laws: possibilities and limitations'. In: Singer, P., Kuhse, H. et al. (Eds). *Embryo Experimentation*. Cambridge: Cambridge University Press.

Gentles, I. (1990). 'The unborn child in civil and criminal law'. *A Time to Choose Life*. London: Stoddart Publishing Co.

Glover, J. (1990). 'Autonomy and rights'. *Causing Death and Saving Lives*. London: Penguin Books.

Green, H.P. (1976). 'The fetus and the law'. In: Milunsky, A., Annas, G.J. (Eds). *Genetics and the Law*. London: Plenum Press.

Grisez, G. (1970). 'Towards a sound public policy'. *Abortion: the Myths, the Realities and the Arguments*. New York: Corpus Books.

Holland, A. (1990). 'A fortnight of my life is missing: a discussion of the status of the human pre embryo'. *Journal of Applied Philosophy,* Vol. 7, No. 1, pp. 25–37.

Kasimba, P. (1990). 'Self regulation and embryo experimentation in Australia: a critique'. In: Singer, P., Kuhse, H. et al. (Eds). *Embryo Experimentation*. Cambridge: Cambridge University Press.

Kelves, D.J., Hood, L. (1993). *The Code of Codes*. USA: Harvard University Press.

Keown, J. (1988). 'The first statutory prohibition of abortion: Lord Ellenborough's Act 1803'. *Abortion, Doctors and the Law: Some Aspects of the Legal Regulation of Abortion in England from 1803–1982.* Cambridge: Cambridge University Press.

Kluge, E-H. (1988). 'When caesarean section operations imposed by the court are justified'. *Journal of Medical Ethics,* Vol. 14, pp. 206–211.

Linden, A.M. (1989). *The Fetus in Law and History Working Paper 58: Crimes Against the Foetus.* Law Reform Commission of Canada.

Mason, J.K., McCall Smith, R.A. (1991). *Law and Medical Ethics.* London: Butterworth and Co.

Meyers, D.W. (1990). 'Mother and fetus: rights in conflict'. *The Human Body and the Law.* Edinburgh: Edinburgh University Press.

Morgan, D. (1992). 'Whatever happened to informed consent?'. *New Law Journal,* 23 October, p. 1448.

Morgan, D., Lee, R.G. (1991). *Blackstone's Guide to the Human Fertilisation and Embryology Act 1990.* London: Blackstone Press Ltd.

Mosher, S. (1993). *A Mother's Ordeal: One Woman's Fight Against China's One Child Policy: The Story of Chi An.* London: Little, Brown & Co.

Office of Population and Census (1995). *Abortion Statistics for 1992 – England and Wales.* London: HMSO.

Pretorius, D. (1993). 'Rights of gametes, zygotes and embryo in storage'. *Medicine and Law,* Vol. 12, pp. 607–616.

Raphael-Leff, J. (1991). 'Pregnancy'. *Psychological Processes of Childbearing.* London: Chapman Hall.

RCOG (1994). *Royal College of Obstetricians and Gynaecologists Guidelines: A Consideration of the Law and Ethics in Relation to Court Authorised Obstetric Intervention.* No. 1, April.

Robertson, J.A. (1989). 'Resolving disputes over frozen embryos'. *The Hastings Centre Report,* November/December, pp. 7–12.

Smith, G.P. (1985-86). 'Australia's frozen "orphan" embryos: a medical, legal and ethical dilemma'. *Journal of Family Law,* Vol. 24, pp. 27–41.

Steinbock, B. (1992a). 'Embryo research and the new reproductive technologies'. *Life Before Birth: The Moral and Legal Status of Embryos and Fetuses.* Oxford: Oxford University Press.

Steinbock, B. (1992b). 'The relevance of illegality'. *The Hastings Centre Reports,* January/February, pp. 19–22.

Walters, L. (1987). 'Ethics and new reproductive technologies: an international review of committee standards'. *The Hastings Centre Report,* Special Supplement, Vol. 17, No. 3, pp. 3–9.

Warnock, M. (1985). *A Question of Life.* Oxford: Basil Blackwell Ltd.

Whitfield, A. (1993). 'Common law duties to unborn children'. *Medical Law Review 1,* January, pp. 28–52.

Wolfenden Report (1957). *Report of the Committee on Homosexual Offences and Prostitution.* Cmnd 247 1957. London: HMSO.

Yates, C.P., Yates, C.B. (1992). 'Fetal rights: sources and implications of an emerging legal concept'. 4th Edition. *Abortion, Medicine and the Law.* Oxford: Facts on File c/o Roundhouse Publishing Co.

Chapter Four

Blair, S.A., Rowan, A. (1990). 'Of mice and men: patents and social policy matters'. *Patent World,* January, pp. 36–38.

Booth, Sir C. (1992). *Our Genetic Future: The Science and Ethics of Genetic Technology* (British Medical Association). Oxford: Oxford University Press.

Brahams, D. (1990). 'Human genetic information: The legal implications'. In: Chadwick, D. et al. (Eds). *Human Genetic Information: Science, Law and Ethics.* Ciba Foundation Symposium 149.

Dixon, P. (1993). *The Genetic Revolution.* Eastbourne: Kingsway Publications.

Family Planning Association (1995). *Contraception: Attitudes and Practice Factsheet No. 3c.* London: Family Planning Association.

Ferguson, M.W.J. (1990). 'Contemporary and future possibilities for human embryonic manipulation'. In: Dyson, A., Harris, J. (Eds). *Experiments on Embryos.* London: Routledge Press.

Glover, J. (1990). *Causing Death and Saving Lives.* London: Penguin Books.

Glover, J. et al. (1989). *Fertility and the Family: The Glover Report on Reproductive Technologies to the European Commission.* London: Fourth Estate Ltd.

Greely, H.T. (1993). 'Health insurance, employment discrimination and the genetic revolution'. In: Kevles, D.J., Hood, L. (Eds). *The Code of Codes.* USA: Harvard University Press.

Harris, J. (1993). *Wonderwoman and Superman: The Ethics of Human Biotechnology.* Oxford: Oxford University Press.

Hoffman, G.M., Karny, G.M. (1988). 'Can justice keep pace with science?'. *Opinion 12 EIPR,* Vol. 12, pp. 354–358.

Holland, A. (1990). 'A fortnight of my life is missing: a discussion of the status of the human pre embryo'. *Journal of Applied Philosophy,* Vol. 7, No. 1, pp. 25–37.

HUFEA (1994, 1995 and 1996). *Human Fertilization and Embryology Authority Annual Reports.* London: Human Fertilization and Embryology Authority.

Jansen, R.P.S. (1985). 'Sperm and ova as property'. *Journal of Medical Ethics,* Vol. 11, pp. 123–126.

Jones, D.G., Telfer, B. (1995). 'Before I was an embryo, I was a pre embryo: or was I?'. *Bioethics,* Vol. 9, No. 1, pp. 32–49.

Kenny, M. (1994). 'The pricking of Father Leo's conscience'. *The Guardian,* 27 October.

Kevles, D.J., Hood, L. (1993). *The Code of Codes.* USA: Harvard University Press.

Mellor, J. (1988). 'Patents and genetic engineering – is it a new problem?'. *Opinion* 6, EIPR, pp. 159–162.

Mihill, C. (1995). 'Mass measles jabs campaign reduces cases to record low'. *The Guardian,* 27 February.

Mihill, C., Ward, D. (1994). 'Vaccination urged by Catholics'. *The Guardian,* 28 October.

Morgan, D., Lee, R.G. (1991). *Blackstone's Guide to the Human Fertilisation and Embryology Act 1990.* London: Blackstone Press Ltd.

Morrow, L. (1991). 'When one body can save another'. *Time Magazine,* 17 June, pp. 44–48.

Nelkin, D. (1993). 'The social power of genetic information'. In: Kewles, D.J., Hood, L. (Eds). *The Code of Codes.* USA: Harvard University Press.

Office of Population and Census (1995). *Abortion Statistics for 1992 – England and Wales.* London: HMSO.

Palmer, J. (1997). 'Europe to allow drug firms to patent genes'. *The Guardian Newspaper,* 16 July.

Phillips, J., Firth, A. (1990). *Introduction to Intellectual Property Law.* London: Butterworths and Co.

Pompidou, A. (1995). 'Research on the human genome and patentability – the ethical consequences'. *Journal of Medical Ethics,* Vol. 21, pp. 69–71.

Silverman, P.H. (1995). 'Commerce and genetic diagnostics'. *Hastings Centre Report Special Supplement,* Vol. 25, No. 3, pp. S15–S18.

Skene, L. (1991). 'Mapping the human genome: some thoughts for those who say "there should be a law on it"'. *Bioethics,* Vol. 5, No. 3, pp. 233–249.

Steinbock, B. (1992). *Life Before Birth: The Moral and Legal Status of Embryos and Fetuses.* Oxford: Oxford University Press.

Ward, K. (1990). 'An irresolvable dispute?'. In: Dyson, A., Harris, J. (Eds). *Experiments on Embryos.* London: Routledge.

Watt, H. (1993). 'Genetic intervention and the good of human beings'. *Catholic Medical Quarterly,* Vol. XLIV, No. 259, pp. 17–21.

Zucker, A. (1992). 'Baby marrow: ethicists and privacy'. *Journal of Medical Ethics,* Vol. 18, pp. 125–127 and 141.

Chapter Five

Berkowitz, J.M. (1995). 'Mummy was a fetus: motherhood and fetal ovarian transplantation'. *Journal of Medical Ethics,* Vol. 21, pp. 298–304.

Braude, P.R. (1992). 'Embryo therapy: what can be done?'. In: Bromham, D. et al. (Eds). *Ethics in Reproductive Medicine.* London: Springler-Verlag.

Ferguson, M.W.J. (1990). 'Contemporary and future possibilities for human embryonic manipulation'. In: Dyson, A., Harris, J. (Eds). *Experiments on Embryos.* London: Routledge Press.

French Anderson, W. (1990). 'Human gene therapy: scientific and ethical considerations'. In: Chadwick, R.F. (Ed). *Ethics, Reproduction and Genetic Control.* London: Routledge Press.

Glover, J. et al. (1989). *Fertility and the Family: The Glover Report on Reproductive Technologies to the European Commission.* London: Fourth Estate Ltd.

Hoskins, B.B., Holmes, H.B. (1984). 'Technology and prenatal femicide'. In: Anditti, R. et al. (Eds). *Test Tube Women: What Future for Motherhood.* London: Pandora Press.

Human Fertilization and Embryology Authority (1995). *In vitro Fertilization* and *Sperm and Egg Donors and the Law.* January. London: HUFEA.

Human Fertilization and Embryology Authority (1996). *Donor Insemination.* March: London: HUFEA.

HUFEA (1994, 1995 and 1996). *Human Fertilization and Embryology Authority Annual Reports.* London: Human Fertilization and Embryology Authority.

Jenkins, R. (1995). *The Law and the Midwife.* Oxford: Blackwell Science Ltd.

Joels, L.A., Wardle, P.G. (1994a). 'Causes and treatments of infertility'. *British Journal of Midwifery Infertility Supplement,* Vol. 2, No. 9, September, pp. 423– 429.

Joels, L.A., Wardle, P.G. (1994b). 'Assisted conception and the midwife'. *British Journal of Midwifery Infertility Supplement,* Vol. 2, No. 9, September, pp. 423– 435.

Kearon, K. (1995). *Medical Ethics: An Introduction.* Dublin, Ireland: Columba Press.

Mason, J.K. (1990). *Medico-Legal Aspects of Reproduction and Parenthood.* Hants, England: Dartmouth Pub. Co. Ltd.

Moore, M. (1996). 'Genetic diagnosis in the first week of gestation'. *Catholic Medical Quarterly*, August, pp. 10–12.

Morgan, D., Lee, R.G. (1991). *Blackstone's Guide to the Human Fertilisation and Embryology Act 1990.* London: Blackstone Press Ltd.

Mosher, S. (1993). *A Mother's Ordeal: One Woman's Fight against China's One Child Policy: The Story of Chi An.* London: Little, Brown & Co.

Rovner, J. (1996). 'US abortion survey produces surprise statistics'. *The Lancet,* Vol. 348, 17th August, p. 469.

Sangari, K. (1984) 'If you would be the mother of a son?'. In: Anditti, R. et al. (Eds). *Test Tube Women: What Future for Motherhood?.* London: Pandora Press.

Smith, S. (1994). 'Moral and ethical issues in infertility treatment'. *British Journal of Midwifery,* Vol. 2, No. 9, September, pp. 436–438.

Steinbock, B. (1992). 'Embryo research and the new reproductive technologies'. *Life Before Birth: The Moral and Legal Status of Embryos and Fetuses.* Oxford: Oxford University Press.

Stern, M., Alton, E. (1996). 'Gene therapy for Cystic Fibrosis'. *Maternal and Child Health,* July/August, pp. 170–173.

Sutton, A. (1993). *Infertility and Assisted Conception: What You Should Know*. London: Catholic Bishops' Joint Committee on Bio-ethical Issues.

Sutton, A. (1996). 'Assisted reproduction: British legislation and some less liberal European approaches'. *Catholic Medical Quarterly*, May, pp. 15–21.

Warwick, C. (1996). 'The Mandy Allwood case: are there questions to be asked?'. *British Journal of Midwifery*, Vol. 4, No. 11, November, pp. 564–65.

Chapter Six

Agar, N. (1995). 'Designing babies: Morally permissible ways to modify the Human Genome'. *Bioethics,* Vol. 9, No. 1, January, pp. 1–31.

Beattie, A. et al. (1993). *Health and Well-Being: A Reader*. London: Macmillan Press Ltd.

Calman, K.C. (1994). *On the State of the Public Health 1993* (Department of Health). London: HMSO.

Downie, R.S. et al. (1990). *Health Promotion: Models and Values*. Oxford: Oxford University Press.

Dixon, P. (1993). *The Genetic Revolution*. Eastbourne: Kingsway Publishers.

Field, M.A. (1989). 'Controlling the woman to protect the fetus'. *Law, Medicine and Health Care,* 17, No. 2, Summer, pp. 114–129.

Green, J.M., Richards, M.P.M. (1993). 'Psychological aspects of fetal screening and the new genetics'. *Journal of Reproductive and Infant Psychology*, Vol. 11, No. 1, January/March.

Holtug, N. (1993). 'Human gene therapy: down the slippery slope?'. *Bioethics,* Vol. 7, No. 5, October, pp. 402–419.

Kevles, D.J., Hood, L. (1993). *The Code of Codes*. USA: Harvard University Press.

Knoppers, B.M. (1993). 'Human genetics: parental, professional and political responsibility'. *Health Law Journal*, Vol. 1, pp. 13–23.

Krimsky, S., Hubbard, R. (1995). 'The business of research'. *Hastings Centre Report*, Vol. 25, No. 1, Jan–Feb, pp. 41–43.

Ledley, F.D. (1994). 'Distinguishing genetics and eugenics on the basis of fairness'. *Journal of Medical Ethics,* Vol. 20, pp. 157–164.

Morgan, D., Lee, R.Ge. (1991). *Blackstone's Guide to the Human Fertilisation and Embryology Act 1990*. London: Blackstone Press Ltd.

Mosher, S. (1993). *A Mother's Ordeal: One Woman's Fight Against China's One Child Policy: The Story of Chi An*. London: Little, Brown & Co.

Office of Population and Census (1995). *Abortion Statistics for 1992 – England and Wales*. London: HMSO.

Resnik, D. (1994). 'Debunking the slippery slope argument against human germ line therapy'. *Journal of Medicine and Philosophy*, Vol. 19, No. 1, February, pp. 23–39.

Richards, M.P.M., Green, J.M. (1993). 'Attitudes towards prenatal screening for fetal abnormality and detection of carriers of genetic disease: a discussion paper'. *Journal of Reproductive and Infant Psychology,* Vol. 11, No. 1, January – March, pp. 49–56.

Schwartz Cowan, R. (1993). 'Genetic technology and choice: an ethics of autonomy'. In: Kevles, D.J., Hood, L. (Eds). *The Code of Codes.* USA: Harvard University Press.

Ward, K. (1990). 'An irresolvable dispute?'. In: Dyson, A., Harris, J. (Eds). *Experiments on Embryos.* London: Routledge.

Watt, H. (1993). 'Genetic intervention and the good of human beings'. *Catholic Medical Quarterly,* Vol. XLIV, No. 259, pp. 17–21.

Webb, P. (1994). 'Some ethical issues in health and patient education'. *Health Promotion and Patient Education: A Professional's Guide.* London: Chapman and Hall.

Index